Pocket reference to renal anemia

Second edition

W0043031

Development of this book was supported by funding from Amgen

Pocket reference to renal anemia
Second edition

Iain C Macdougall, BSc, MD, FRCP
Consultant Nephrologist and Professor of Clinical Nephrology
Department of Renal Medicine
King's College Hospital
London, UK

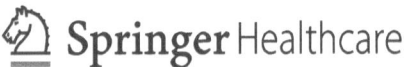

Published by Springer Healthcare Ltd, 236 Gray's Inn Road, London, WC1X 8HB, UK.

www.springerhealthcare.com

© 2013 Springer Healthcare, a part of Springer Science+Business Media.

First edition 2003
Second edition 2013

British Library Cataloguing-in-Publication Data.

A catalogue record for this book is available from the British Library.

ISBN 978 1 908517 74 6

Project editor: Alla Zarifyan
Designer: Joe Harvey
Artworker: Sissan Mollerfors
Production: Marina Maher
Printed in Great Britain by Latimer Trend

Contents

Dedication		**vii**
Author biography		**ix**
1	**What is renal anemia?**	**1**
	References	4
2	**What is the cause of renal anemia?**	**5**
	Erythropoietin deficiency	5
	Uremic inhibitors	7
	Inflammation	7
	Hepcidin	9
	Iron deficiency	10
	Hyperparathyroidism	10
	Aluminum toxicity	11
	Shortened red blood cell life span	12
	References	12
3	**Stepwise approach to anemia management in patients with chronic kidney disease**	**13**
	Step 1: Exclude other causes of anemia	14
	Step 2: Iron management	14
	Step 3: Erythropoiesis-stimulating agent therapy	14
	Step 4: Blood transfusions	14
	References	14
4	**Excluding other causes of anemia**	**15**
	Reticulocyte count	17
	References	19

5 Iron management   **21**

Iron deficiency: absolute versus functional   21

Detection of iron deficiency   22

Iron supplementation: oral versus intravenous   24

References   27

6 Erythropoiesis-stimulating agent therapy   **29**

Epoetins (including "biosimilars")   29

Darbepoetin alfa   30

Methoxypolyethylene glycol epoetin beta   30

Peginesatide   31

Normal Hematocrit Trial, CREATE, CHOIR, and TREAT   32

Trigger hemoglobin concentration   34

Target hemoglobin   34

Erythropoiesis-stimulating agent therapy and the risk of malignancy   35

Erythropoiesis-stimulating agent therapy and the risk of stroke   36

Poor response to erythropoiesis-stimulating agent therapy   38

Adjuvant therapy   41

References   41

7 Blood transfusions   **45**

References   47

8 Guidelines on the management of renal anemia   **49**

References   51

9 What is the future of renal anemia management?   **53**

Hypoxia-inducible factor stabilizers   53

Hepcidin modulation   54

Other strategies   55

References   55

10 Conclusions   **57**

Dos and don'ts in renal anemia management   **58**

Learning points   **59**

References   61

Dedication

Dedicated to my parents, Mary and Alasdair, my lovely wife, Penny, and our six children, Jennifer, Alan, Daniel, Inigo, Ella, and Nancy.

Author biography

Iain C Macdougall is Consultant Nephrologist (from January 1996) and Professor of Clinical Nephrology (from September 2010) at King's College Hospital, London. His undergraduate training was obtained from Glasgow University, Scotland, from which he was awarded a First Class Honours BSc in Pharmacology in 1980, and his medical degree in 1983. Professor Macdougall then completed his general medical and nephrology training at hospitals in Glasgow, Cardiff, and London. He developed a research interest in renal anemia while a clinical research fellow in Cardiff (1988–1991) and extended this interest during his appointment at St Bartholomew's Hospital (1991–1996), where he studied the potential role of proinflammatory cytokines in mediating resistance to epoetin.

Professor Macdougall has been involved in numerous advisory boards in renal anemia management worldwide, including the Working Parties responsible for both the 1999 and the 2004 versions of the European Best Practice Guidelines, along with the Work Group that produced the US KDOQI Guidelines on Renal Anemia Management (2006; update 2007) and the recently published global KDIGO Anemia Guidelines (August 2012). He was a previous board member of the KDIGO initiative, and a council member of the European Renal Association from 2004 until 2007. He has been the UK lead on several pivotal clinical trials of anemia management in patients with chronic kidney disease, including CREATE and TREAT, and he chairs the Anaemia Clinical Study Group of the UK Kidney Research Consortium. He is frequently invited to lecture both nationally and internationally on this topic, and he has coauthored the section on renal anemia for the last three editions of the *Oxford Textbook of Clinical Nephrology*.

Chapter 1

What is renal anemia?

Anemia is defined as a reduction in the number of red blood cells (RBCs) in the blood, most accurately assessed by measuring the RBC mass using isotopic dilution methods. However, such blood volume studies are neither practical nor cost effective for routine clinical use in patients and, as a result, anemia is usually defined as a reduction in one or more of the major RBC measurements: hemoglobin concentration, hematocrit, or RBC count.

- *Hemoglobin* is a heme-containing protein, whose physiological function is to carry oxygen around the body. Values are usually expressed as grams of hemoglobin per 100 mL of whole blood (g/dL).
- *Hematocrit* is the percentage of a volume of whole blood that is occupied by intact RBCs.
- *RBC count* is the number of RBCs contained in a unit of whole blood. Values are usually expressed as millions of RBCs per μL of whole blood (or x 10^{12}/L).

The normal ranges for these and other RBC parameters are shown in Table 1.1. Based on statistics from the general population [2], anemia is defined as a hemoglobin level more than two standard deviations below the mean; this is approximately <13.0 g/dL in men and approximately <12.0 g/dL in women (as defined by the World Health Organization nearly half a century ago) [2]. Some of the older literature on anemia tends to use the term "hematocrit" rather than "hemoglobin" as a measure of this condition; however, this is now regarded as bad practice, due to

I. C. Macdougall, *Pocket Reference to Renal Anemia*,
DOI: 10.1007/978-1-907673-48-1_1, © Springer Healthcare 2013

Normal values for red blood cell parameters

RBC parameter	Adult men	Adult women
Hemoglobin (g/dL)	15.7 ± 1.7	13.8 ± 1.5
Hematocrit (%)	46.0 ± 4.0	40.0 ± 4.0
RBC count (x10^{12}/L)	5.2 ± 0.7	4.6 ± 0.5
Reticulocytes (%)	1.6 ± 0.5	1.4 ± 0.5
MCV (fL)	88.0 ± 8.0	88.0 ± 8.0
MCH (pg)	30.4 ± 2.8	30.4 ± 2.8
MCHC (g/dL)	34.4 ± 1.1	34.4 ± 1.1
RDW (%)	13.1 ± 1.4	13.1 ± 1.4

Table 1.1 Normal values for red blood cell parameters. Values given include 95% confidence limits. MCH, mean cell hemoglobin; MCHC, mean cell hemoglobin concentration; MCV, mean corpuscular volume; RBC, red blood cell; RDW, red cell volume distribution width. Adapted with permission from Beutler et al [1].

the many external factors influencing hematocrit, as well as the lack of an international standard for this measurement.

There is no absolute cut-off to define anemia in patients with chronic kidney disease (CKD). In this patient population, an arbitrary definition of anemia was a hemoglobin concentration <11 g/dL, based on previous guidelines for triggering the use of erythropoiesis-stimulating agent (ESA) therapy [3].

Anemia is a highly prevalent complication in patients with CKD, occurring in around 5% of patients with CKD stage 3, and increasing to over 90% of patients on chronic dialysis [4]. It is associated with a number of adverse outcomes, including death and nonfatal cardiovascular events, and it also has an adverse effect on patients' physical capacities and quality of life. Furthermore, anemic CKD patients show an increased requirement for RBC transfusions compared to those whose anemia is corrected.

"Renal" anemia is defined as a chronic anemia in which the circulating plasma erythropoietin levels are inappropriately low for the degree of anemia [5]. This usually occurs when the glomerular filtration rate (GFR) falls below 30 mL/min (corresponding to a serum creatinine level of approximately 300 μmol/L), although the US National Health and Nutrition Examination Survey (NHANES 3) data suggested that mild degrees of anemia may be present with a GFR of up to 60 mL/min [6], and indeed diabetics appear to develop inappropriately low levels of

erythropoietin at a higher GFR cut-off compared to nondiabetics. Thus, it is not uncommon for diabetic subjects to develop renal anemia when their GFR falls below 45 mL/min [7].

Learning point 1
Renal anemia usually occurs when the GFR falls below 30 mL/min, although mild degrees of anemia may be present with a GFR of up to 60 mL/min [6].

Learning point 2
Diabetics appear to develop inappropriately low levels of erythropoietin at a higher GFR cut-off compared to nondiabetics. Thus it is not uncommon for diabetic subjects to develop renal anemia when their GFR falls below 45 mL/min [7].

Erythropoietin is a glycoprotein hormone, which is produced in the kidneys, and is responsible for maintaining the RBC count at a constant level of approximately 5×10^{12}/L [8]. In healthy individuals under normal circumstances, the bone marrow manufactures approximately 120 million new RBCs every minute, and this compensates for the obligatory loss of RBCs from the circulation. The RBC count is usually maintained at a constant level, although the absolute level differs among individuals within the same gender by as much as 15% [9]. In general, men have higher hemoglobin levels than women, due to a greater production of testosterone. In premenopausal women, this is exacerbated by the monthly loss of RBCs due to menstruation.

Learning point 3
In healthy individuals, the bone marrow manufactures approximately 120 million new RBCs every minute.

There are many causes of anemia, including blood loss, hemolysis, and iron deficiency, but a classification of "renal anemia" requires the patient to have inappropriately low plasma levels of erythropoietin

(Figure 1.1) [5]. By the definitions described here, significant anemia may be present in up to 90% of patients on dialysis, and up to 67% of patients starting regular dialysis [4].

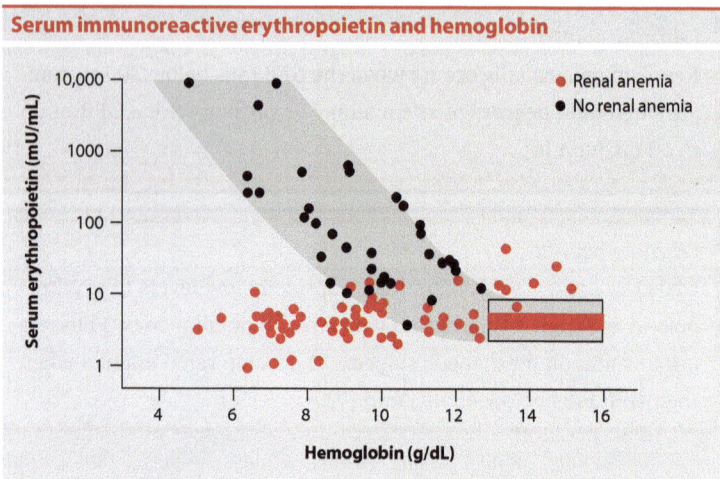

Serum immunoreactive erythropoietin and hemoglobin

Figure 1.1 Serum immunoreactive erythropoietin and hemoglobin. The graph represents the relationship between serum immunoreactive erythropoietin levels and hemoglobin concentration in nonrenal anemia and in patients with chronic kidney disease (excluding those with polycystic kidneys). The rectangle indicates the interquartile range and 95% confidence range of erythropoietin levels in nonanemic healthy adults. Adapted from Macdougall [10].

References

1   Beutler E, Lichtman LA, Coller BS, et al. *Williams Hematology*. 5th edn. New York, USA: McGraw-Hill; 1995.
2   World Health Organization. Nutritional Anaemias: Report of a WHO Scientific Group. Geneva, Switzerland: World Health Organization; 1968.
3   Locatelli F, Aljama P, Barany P, et al. Revised European best practice guidelines for the management of anaemia in patients with chronic renal failure. *Nephrol Dial Transplant*. 2004;19(suppl 2):ii1-47.
4   Pereira BJG. New perspectives in chronic renal insufficiency. *Am J Kidney Dis*. 2000;36(suppl 3):S1-S3.
5   Caro J, Brown S, Miller O, et al. Erythropoietin levels in uremic nephric and anephric patients. *J Lab Clin Med*. 1979;93:449-458.
6   Astor BC, Muntner P, Levin A, et al. Association of kidney function with anemia: the Third National Health and Nutrition Examination Survey (1988–1994). *Arch Intern Med*. 2002;162:1401-1408.
7   Thomas MC, MacIsaac RJ, Tsalamandris C, Power D, Jerums G. Unrecognized anemia in patients with diabetes: a cross-sectional survey. *Diabetes Care*. 2003;26:1164-1169.
8   Fisher JW. Erythropoietin: physiology and pharmacology update. *Exp Biol Med*. 2003;228:1-14.
9   Mayo Clinic. Complete blood count (CBC). www.mayoclinic.com/health/complete-blood-count/MY00476/DSECTION=results. Updated August 10, 2012. Accessed February 6, 2013.
10 Macdougall IC. Anaemia and chronic renal failure. *Medicine*. 2011;39:425-428.

Development of this book was supported by funding from Amgen

Chapter 2

What is the cause of renal anemia?

The pathogenesis of renal anemia is multifactorial, with a number of contributory processes involved, to a greater or lesser extent.

Erythropoietin deficiency

As discussed in Chapter 1, the major cause of renal anemia is a relative deficiency of erythropoietin from the kidneys [1]. Erythropoietin is a single-chain, polypeptide hormone with a molecular weight of 30.4 kDa. Approximately 40% of the molecule is carbohydrate in the form of three N-linked glycosylation chains and one O-linked glycosylation chain (Figure 2.1) [2]. The erythropoietin gene is located on chromosome 7, and there is minimal post-translational modification [3,4].

Erythropoietin is synthesized in the peritubular interstitial cells of the kidneys, and a small amount is also produced in the liver. There are no preformed stores of erythropoietin, and the production of this hormone is stimulated by hypoxia (Figure 2.2). It was previously believed that the reason for inappropriately low circulating erythropoietin levels in patients with CKD was that the main cells in the body producing erythropoietin were damaged by the same process that was causing the renal failure. Recently, however, it became clear that with an appropriate stimulus (eg, hypoxia, or a mimic of hypoxia caused by pharmacological stabilization of hypoxia-inducible factor [HIF], the main transcription factor for the erythropoietin gene; see Chapter 9), patients with end-stage renal failure are still able to increase their plasma concentrations of

I. C. Macdougall, *Pocket Reference to Renal Anemia*,
DOI: 10.1007/978-1-907673-48-1_2, © Springer Healthcare 2013

Structure of erythropoietin

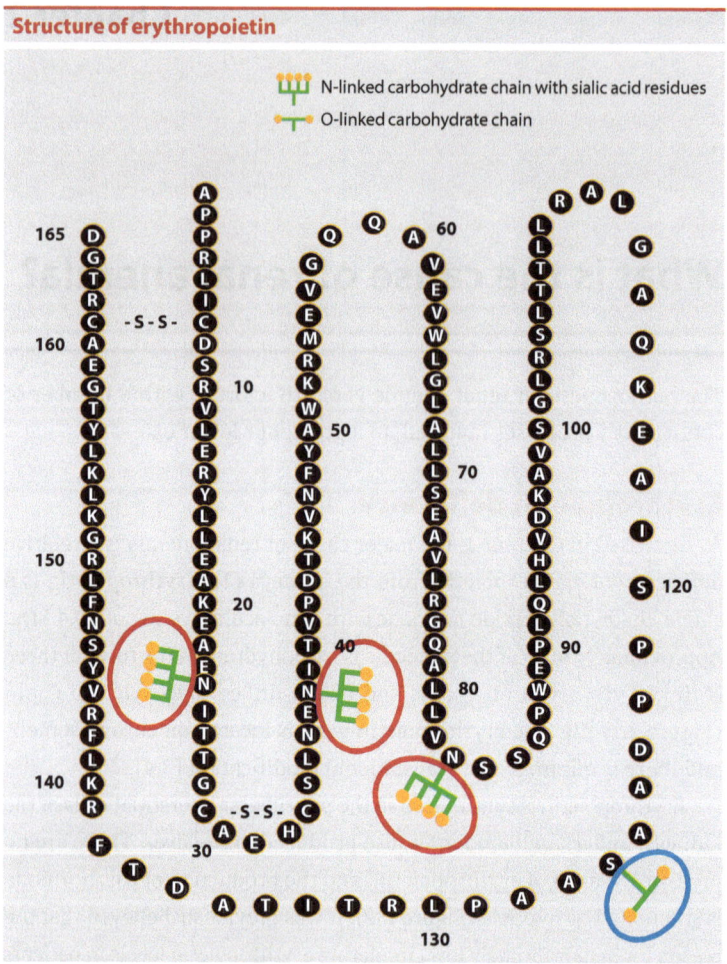

Figure 2.1 Structure of erythropoietin.

erythropoietin [5]. Indeed, even anephric individuals are able to show some response, and in this context it is believed that erythropoietin is probably being produced by liver cells, which are known to possess mRNA for the protein [5]. Thus, the inappropriately low erythropoietin production in patients with end-stage renal failure may be partly related to loss of the kidney cells synthesizing the hormone, but also partly due to a malfunction of the oxygen-sensing stimulus.

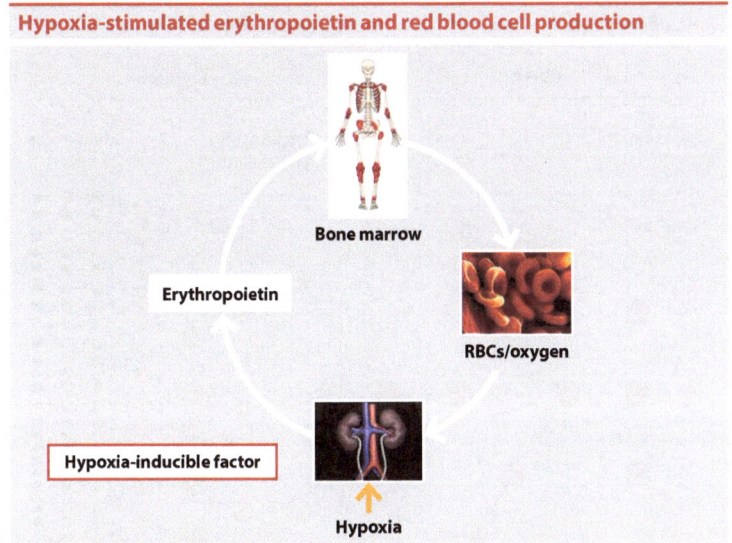

Hypoxia-stimulated erythropoietin and red blood cell production

Bone marrow

Erythropoietin

RBCs/oxygen

Hypoxia-inducible factor

Hypoxia

Figure 2.2 Hypoxia-stimulated erythropoietin and red blood cell production.
RBC, red blood cells.

In the absence of anemia or hypoxia, the plasma erythropoietin level is normally very constant in any given individual. Erythropoietin acts on erythroid progenitor cells in the bone marrow, preventing their apoptosis and allowing them to proliferate (Figure 2.3). The normal range of plasma erythropoietin is around 4–30 mU/mL, but levels 100–1000 times higher may be found in several nonrenal causes of anemia [1].

Uremic inhibitors

In the 1970s, it was recognized that uremic serum inhibited erythroid colony growth (Figure 2.4). Prior to the advent of recombinant human erythropoietin, it was believed that several substances in uremic serum could inhibit erythropoiesis [7], including spermine, spermidine, putrescine, cadaverine, and parathyroid hormone.

Inflammation

Uremia is now recognized to be a chronic inflammatory state, and at least part of the pathogenesis of renal anemia is similar to the pathogenesis of the anemia of chronic inflammation. Proinflammatory cytokines,

Role of erythropoietin in red blood cell development

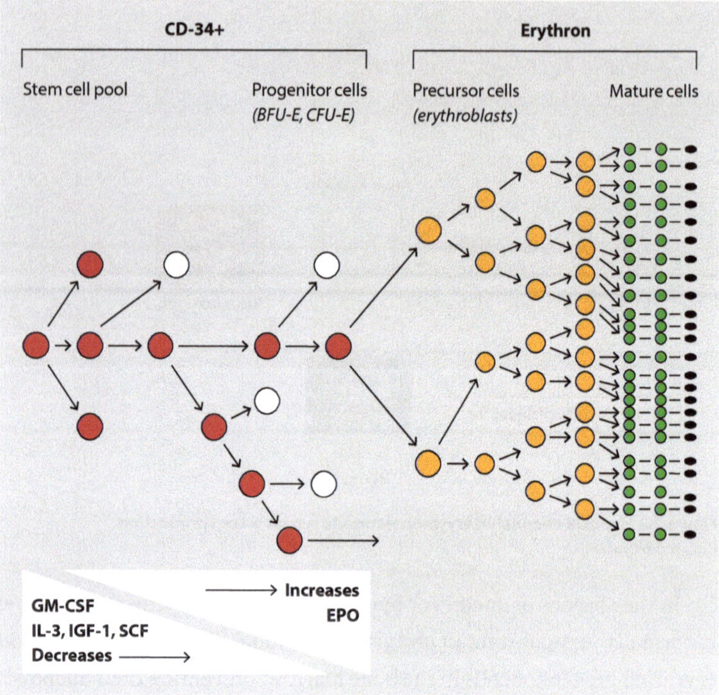

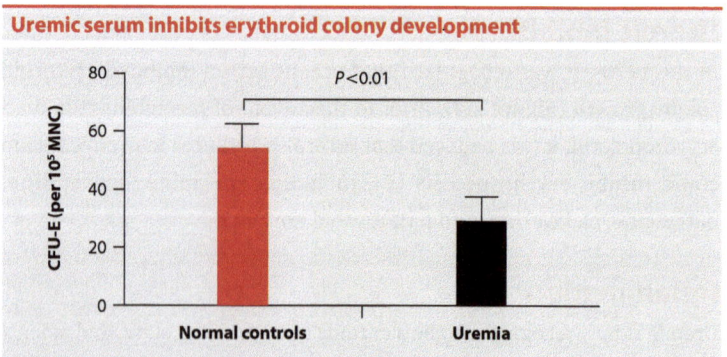

Figure 2.3 Role of erythropoietin in red blood cell development. BFU-E, burst-forming units – erythroid; CFU-E, colony-forming units – erythroid; EPO, erythropoietin; GM-CSF, granulocyte–macrophage colony-stimulating factor; IL-3, interleukin-3; IGF-1, insulin-like growth factor-1; SCF, stem cell factor.

Uremic serum inhibits erythroid colony development

Figure 2.4 Uremic serum inhibits erythroid colony development. CFU-E, colony-forming units – erythroid; MNC, mononuclear cells. Adapted with permission from Allen et al [6].

such as tumor necrosis factor alfa and interferon gamma may also play a part in causing suppression of erythropoiesis in renal failure. Removal of such substances by increasing the dialysis prescription may improve erythropoiesis in renal patients [8]. In addition, it is now recognized that hepcidin, the master regulator of iron homeostasis in the body, also plays a major role in inflammatory anemia, by limiting iron availability to the bone marrow. Hepcidin is upregulated by proinflammatory cytokines, particularly interleukin-6 (IL-6) [9].

Hepcidin

Hepcidin is a 25-amino-acid peptide, which is produced in the liver in response to a number of stimuli, including inflammation and iron overload. The regulation of hepcidin is beginning to be understood, and certain factors such as hemojuvelin and bone morphogenetic protein-6 are implicated in its production in hepatocytes and macrophages. Its principal physiological role is to regulate the amount of iron available to the bone marrow for erythropoiesis by acting on enterocytes in the duodenum to limit iron absorption from the gut, as well as iron release from hepatocytes, macrophages, and splenic cells (Figure 2.5) [10]. Its main action is to bind to ferroportin, the sole cellular exporter of iron

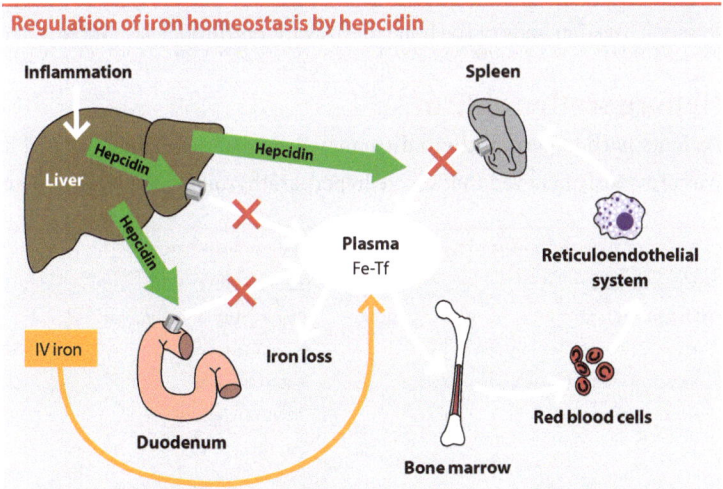

Figure 2.5 Regulation of iron homeostasis by hepcidin. Fe-Tf, iron–transferrin complex.

in mammals. Patients with CKD, particularly those on hemodialysis, are known to have high circulating levels of hepcidin, and this is partly due to their chronic inflammatory state, and partly due to reduced clearance of hepcidin via the kidneys [11].

Iron deficiency

Patients with CKD are often in negative iron balance due to a combination of low dietary intake of iron as well as increased iron losses. The low dietary intake of iron is caused by poor appetite in patients with uremia, and by poor absorption from the gut due to hepcidin upregulation. Certain drugs may also inhibit iron absorption such as proton pump inhibitors and phosphate binders. Also, certain foods, such as tea can have the same effect.

Increased iron losses are due to a number of factors, including platelet dysfunction secondary to uremia and increased mucosal inflammation and ulceration in the gastrointestinal tract, the use of anticoagulants such as heparin on dialysis, and the use of aspirin and antiplatelet drugs in cardiovascular prophylaxis (Table 2.1) [12]. Iron losses in hemodialysis patients are known to be up to 5 or 6 times higher than those of normal healthy individuals [13]. There are two types of iron deficiency: absolute, when the total body stores of iron are exhausted, and functional, when there are adequate or increased stores of iron, but an inability to release the iron rapidly enough to satisfy the demands of the bone marrow for erythropoiesis (Table 2.2).

Hyperparathyroidism

Patients with hyperparathyroidism may become anemic, and indeed it was previously believed that severe hyperparathyroidism may exacerbate

Causes of iron deficiency in patients with chronic kidney disease	
Reduced intake	**Increased loss**
Poor appetite	Occult gastrointestinal losses
Poor gastrointestinal absorption	Peptic ulceration
Concurrent medication (eg, omeprazole)	Blood sampling
Food interactions	Dialysis losses
	Concurrent medications (eg, aspirin)
	Heparin on dialysis

Table 2.1 Causes of iron deficiency in patients with chronic kidney disease.

Definition of absolute and functional iron deficiency	
Absolute	Reduced body iron stores
	Low serum ferritin levels
Functional	Normal body iron stores, but a failure to release iron rapidly enough to satisfy demands of bone marrow
	Normal/high serum ferritin
	↓ Transferrin saturation (<20%)
	↑ Hypochromic red blood cells (>10%)

Table 2.2 Definition of absolute and functional iron deficiency.

renal anemia. Several mechanisms were proposed to account for this effect, including the development of fibrosis in the bone marrow (a condition known as osteitis fibrosa cystica), along with direct suppression of erythroid colony growth by parathyroid hormone. In the absence of bone marrow fibrosis, hyperparathyroidism per se contributes little to the development of renal anemia, as this can easily be overcome by recombinant human erythropoietin therapy. Nevertheless, some patients with resistance to this treatment have shown enhanced erythropoietic activity after parathyroidectomy (Figure 2.6) [14].

Aluminum toxicity

In previous times, this was an important contributory factor in the pathogenesis of renal anemia. The anemia was characteristically microcytic

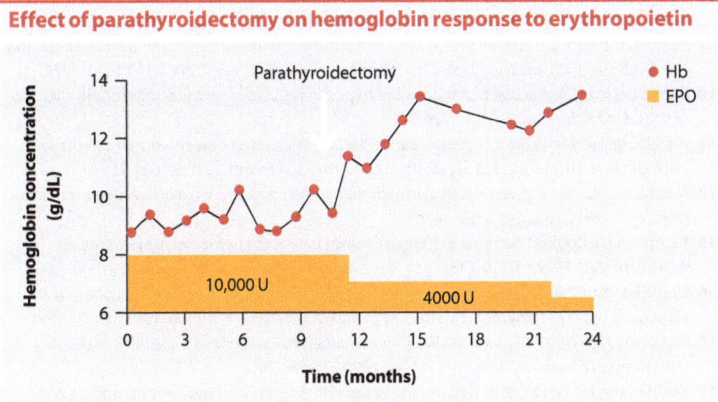

Effect of parathyroidectomy on hemoglobin response to erythropoietin

Figure 2.6 Effect of parathyroidectomy on hemoglobin response to erythropoietin.
Hb, hemoglobin; EPO, erythropoietin.

in origin, even in the absence of iron deficiency. With the introduction of improved water purification and deionization, and the decreased use of aluminum-containing phosphate-binders, aluminum toxicity no longer occurs. It was previously treated with intravenous desferrioxamine on dialysis [15].

Shortened red blood cell life span

The life span of an RBC in normal healthy individuals is approximately 120 days. RBC survival studies in uremic patients have indicated that the average life span of an RBC is generally shorter than this, as low as 60–90 days; this is due to increased RBC fragility, causing low-grade hemolysis [16,17].

References

1 Caro J, Brown S, Miller O, et al. Erythropoietin levels in uremic nephric and anephric patients. *J Lab Clin Med*. 1979;93:449-458.
2 Fisher JW. Erythropoietin: physiology and pharmacology update. *Exp Biol Med*. 2003;228:1-14.
3 Lai PH, Everett R, Wang FF, et al. Structural characterization of human erythropoietin. *J Biol Chem*. 1986;261:3116-3121.
4 Browne JK, Cohen AM, Egrie JC. Erythropoietin: gene cloning protein structure and biological properties. *Cold Spring Harbor Symp Quant Biol*. 1986;51:693-702.
5 Bernhardt WM, Wiesener MS, Scigalla P, et al. Inhibition of prolyl hydroxylases increases erythropoietin production in ESRD. *J Am Soc Nephrol*. 2010;21:2151-2156.
6 Allen DA, Breen C, Yaqoob MM, Macdougall IC. Inhibition of CFU-E colony formation in uremic patients with inflammatory disease: role of IFN-γ and TNF-α. *J Investig Med*. 1999;47:204-211.
7 Macdougall IC. Role of uremic toxins in exacerbating anemia in renal failure. *Kidney Int Suppl*. 2001;78: S67-S72.
8 Ifudu O, Feldman J, Friedman EA. The intensity of hemodialysis and the response to erythropoietin in patients with end-stage renal disease. *N Engl J Med*. 1996;334:420-425.
9 Nemeth E, Rivera S, Gabayan V, et al. IL-6 mediates hypoferremia of inflammation by inducing the synthesis of the iron regulatory hormone hepcidin. *J Clin Invest*. 2004;113:1271-1276.
10 Babitt JL, Lin HY. Molecular mechanisms of hepcidin regulation: implications for the anemia of CKD. *Am J Kidney Dis*. 2010;55:726-741.
11 Macdougall IC, Malyszko J, Hider RC, Bansal SS. Current status of the measurement of blood hepcidin levels in chronic kidney disease. *Clin J Am Soc Nephrol*. 2010;5:1681-1689.
12 Macdougall IC. Iron supplementation in nephrology and oncology: what do we have in common? *Oncologist*. 2011;16(suppl 3):25-34.
13 Eschbach JW, Cook JD, Scribner BH, Finch CA. Iron balance in hemodialysis patients. *Ann Intern Med*. 1977;87:710-713.
14 Ureña P, Eckardt KU, Sarfati E, et al. Serum erythropoietin and erythropoiesis in primary and secondary hyperparathyroidism: effect of parathyroidectomy. *Nephron*. 1991;59:384-393.
15 McCarthy JT, Milliner DS, Johnson WJ. Clinical experience with desferrioxamine in dialysis patients with aluminium toxicity. *Q J Med*. 1990;74:257-276.
16 Wu SG, Jeng FR, Wei SY, et al. Red blood cell osmotic fragility in chronically hemodialyzed patients. *Nephron*. 1998;78:28-32.
17 Vos FE, Schollum JB, Coulter CV, Doyle TC, Duffull SB, Walker RJ. Red blood cell survival in long-term dialysis patients. *Am J Kidney Dis*. 2011;58:591-598.

Development of this book was supported by funding from Amgen

Chapter 3

Stepwise approach to anemia management in patients with chronic kidney disease

Broadly speaking, a pragmatic approach to anemia management in patients with CKD should follow a stepwise approach using four steps (Figure 3.1) [1].

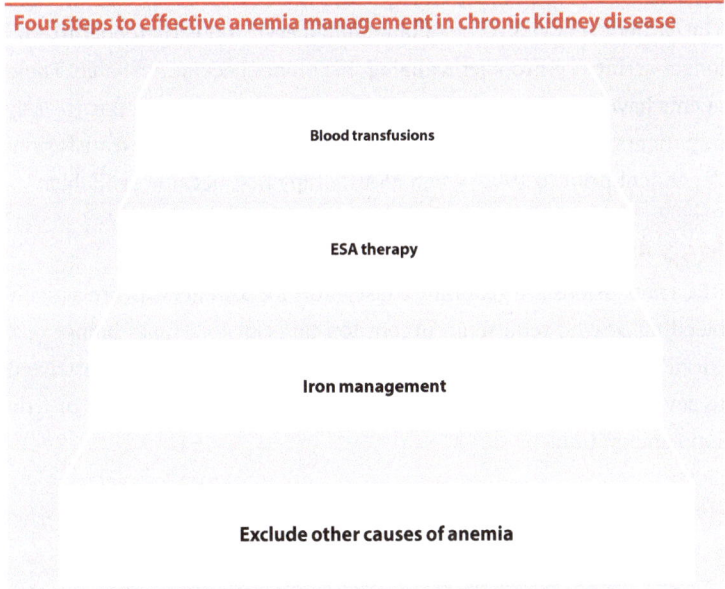

Four steps to effective anemia management in chronic kidney disease

Blood transfusions

ESA therapy

Iron management

Exclude other causes of anemia

Figure 3.1 Four steps to effective anemia management in chronic kidney disease.
ESA, erythropoiesis-stimulating agent.

I. C. Macdougall, *Pocket Reference to Renal Anemia*,
DOI: 10.1007/978-1-907673-48-1_3, © Springer Healthcare 2013

Step 1: Exclude other causes of anemia

Although the major cause of anemia associated with CKD is inappropriately low circulating erythropoietin levels, there are many other causes of anemia, and these should be excluded before any consideration is given to using ESA therapy.

Step 2: Iron management

Iron deficiency is also an important contributory cause of anemia in renal patients, and this too should be investigated and treated in any CKD patient found to be anemic. Intravenous iron therapy is widely used in the CKD population, particularly in hemodialysis patients where iron losses are unable to be matched by dietary or oral iron supplementation.

Step 3: Erythropoiesis-stimulating agent therapy

Most patients with CKD anemia have inappropriately low erythropoietin levels, and it is logical to replace this with supplemental ESA therapy. The earlier agent was recombinant human erythropoietin (epoetin), and longer-acting erythropoietin analogs have since become available. These agents have transformed the management of CKD anemia, particularly in patients on hemodialysis, many of whom were heavily transfusion-dependent prior to 1990, when ESA therapy first became available.

Step 4: Blood transfusions

RBC transfusions are generally a last resort for patients who are actively bleeding or who require an urgent top-up prior to a renal biopsy or a surgical procedure. Their role in chronic anemia should be restricted to severe symptomatic anemia unresponsive to ESA therapy or iron supplementation.

References

1   National Kidney Foundation. KDIGO clinical practice guideline for anemia in chronic kidney disease. *Kidney Int Suppl.* 2012;2:v-335.

Development of this book was supported by funding from Amgen

Chapter 4

Excluding other causes of anemia

Data from the NHANES 3 provide helpful information on the expected mean hemoglobin at various stages of CKD development [1]. Anemia is uncommon in CKD stages 1 and 2, starts to develop in early stage 3, and becomes highly prevalent in late stage 3, and stages 4 and 5 (Figure 4.1). The vast majority of patients on chronic dialysis are anemic to a greater or lesser extent. Thus, CKD patients in stages 1, 2, and early stage 3, who are found to be anemic, require stringent investigations for other causes of anemia, as renal anemia alone is much less likely [1].

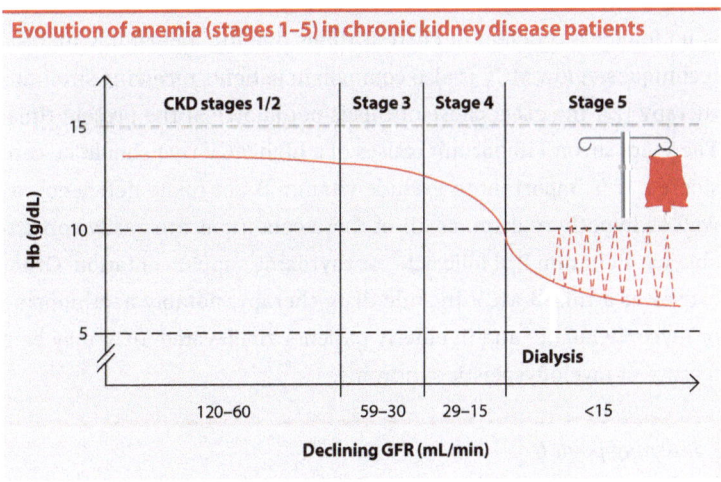

Evolution of anemia (stages 1–5) in chronic kidney disease patients

Figure 4.1 Evolution of anemia (stages 1–5) in chronic kidney disease patients. CKD, chronic kidney disease; GFR, glomerular filtration rate; Hb, hemoglobin.

I. C. Macdougall, *Pocket Reference to Renal Anemia*,
DOI: 10.1007/978-1-907673-48-1_4, © Springer Healthcare 2013

> *Learning point 4*
> CKD patients in stages 1, 2, and early stage 3, who are found to be anemic, require stringent investigations for other causes of anemia, as renal anemia alone is much less likely [1].

"Pure" renal anemia is usually normochromic and normocytic, and either a low or high mean corpuscular volume (MCV), or low mean cell hemoglobin (MCH) or mean cell hemoglobin concentration (MCHC) strongly suggest other contributory causes.

> *Learning point 5*
> "Pure" renal anemia is usually normochromic and normocytic, and either a low or high MCV, or low MCH or MCHC strongly suggest other contributory causes.

Examination of the blood cell indices and white cell and platelet counts may be helpful. In previous times, a low MCV was suggestive of aluminum overload, either through poor-quality dialysis or the use of aluminum-containing phosphate binders. Aluminum overload is no longer a problem in current times due to modern-day dialysis techniques. A low MCV is also common in patients receiving sirolimus therapy [2]; the exact cause of this is not known at the present time. There are several important causes of a high MCV that should be considered. It is important to exclude vitamin B_{12} or folate deficiency, as well as hypothyroidism, as all of these conditions are easily correctable with vitamin B_{12}, folic acid, or thyroxine supplementation. Other causes of a raised MCV include drug therapy, notably azathioprine or mycophenolate, and in elderly patients an elevated MCV may be a feature of myelodysplastic syndrome.

> *Learning point 6*
> A low MCV commonly occurs in patients receiving sirolimus therapy [2].

In patients of certain ethnic background (eg, Africans have a relatively high rate of sickle cell anemia and natives of some Mediterranean countries such as Greece have a higher rate of thalassemia), hemoglobin electrophoresis should be performed to ascertain whether or not the patient has a hemoglobinopathy. In progressive iron deficiency, RBCs will become hypochromic and deficient in intracellular hemoglobin before the MCV becomes abnormal. A decreased MCH or MCHC therefore indicates longstanding iron deficiency; if a low MCV is also evident, then this suggests an even longer exposure to iron deficiency.

Learning point 7
A low MCV coupled with a low MCH or MCHC indicates either iron deficiency or a hemoglobinopathy.

A sudden change in MCV or other RBC parameters (such as RBC distribution width) suggest that the patient may have been transfused. This is the only possible cause of a rapid increase or decrease in MCV, as well as a sharp rise in RBC width, both suggesting more than one population of circulating RBCs.

Learning point 8
A rapid change in MCV and/or RBC volume distribution width strongly suggest that the patient has had a recent RBC transfusion.

Abnormalities of white cell count or platelet count suggest an underlying hematological disorder, which may justify a bone marrow examination if there is no other obvious cause.

Reticulocyte count

Previously, reticulocytes were counted under the microscope on a blood film. This was not only laborious for the hematology technician, but was also very inaccurate. Modern-day automated blood count analyzers allow for a very accurate reticulocyte count, and this is usually expressed in two ways: (i) absolute count or (ii) percentage of reticulocytes in the total RBC population. The absolute count is generally more helpful, and a normal reticulocyte count in healthy individuals is generally above 50 x 10^9/L. CKD patients may run reticulocyte counts of around 30 x 10^9–60 x 10^9/L, although clearly this will be higher if the patient is receiving ESA therapy. Reticulocyte counts lower than 40 x 10^9/L on ESA therapy suggest a degree of bone marrow failure, and low reticulocyte counts may suggest a need for a bone marrow examination. Very low reticulocyte counts of less than 10 x 10^9/L suggest severe bone marrow failure, such that occurs with antibody-mediated pure red cell aplasia or aplastic anemia [3]. Antibody-mediated pure red cell aplasia is a complication of ESA therapy, caused by antibodies developing against the ESA that cross-react with endogenous erythropoietin, effectively shutting down RBC production in the bone marrow. The condition is confirmed on bone marrow examination where absence or near-absence of erythroid progenitor cells in the bone marrow is evident. Circulating anti-erythropoietin antibodies may be detectable by immunoassay and the patient is often transfusion-dependent [3].

> *Learning point 9*
> A reticulocyte count of <10 x 10^9/L suggests severe bone marrow failure, possibly due to antibody-mediated pure red cell aplasia or another hematological condition [3].

Higher reticulocyte counts (eg, >100 x 10^9/L) suggest an active bone marrow, but in the presence of anemia this indicates enhanced RBC loss, due to either hemolysis or bleeding.

> *Learning point 10*
> Reticulocyte counts of >100 x 10^9/L suggest an active bone marrow but enhanced RBC loss, due to either hemolysis or bleeding.

CKD patients are also prone to a number of acute and chronic inflammatory conditions, and a raised C-reactive protein level may potentially suggest an underlying infective or inflammatory cause. Other clues may be a low serum albumin level or high ferritin level, as both of these laboratory parameters are influenced as part of the acute phase response.

A well-recognized, but often ignored, cause of chronic inflammation is a failed kidney transplant, still *in situ*, which may potentially harbor a massive pool of proinflammatory cytokines [4].

A detailed history for possible causes of blood loss should be taken, and there may be a need for an upper gastrointestinal endoscopy, colonoscopy, or even small bowel video capsule enteroscopy. A low ferritin level, particularly if this persists despite repeated top-up injections of intravenous iron, may provide additional criteria for subjecting the patient to more detailed gastrointestinal investigations.

If hemolysis is suspected, then a blood film may be useful to detect RBC fragments. A positive Coombs test may indicate an immune-mediated hemolysis, whilst a raised bilirubin or lactate dehydrogenase level would also be consistent with a hemolytic process. A low serum haptoglobin level would also suggest underlying hemolysis. Thus, any patient who does not appear to be bleeding, but who has a high reticulocyte count and/or a normal or high ferritin level should be assessed for underlying hemolysis by measuring bilirubin levels, lactate dehydrogenase, serum haptoglobins, a blood film, and Coombs test.

In certain circumstances, other, more specialist, tests of causes of both renal impairment and anemia may be helpful (eg, myeloma may induce both kidney and bone marrow disease, causing renal dysfunction and anemia together). Thus, serum electrophoresis looking for a paraprotein and/or measurement of serum free light chains may be indicated.

References

1   Astor BC, Muntner P, Levin A, et al. Association of kidney function with anemia: the Third National Health and Nutrition Examination Survey (1988–1994). *Arch Intern Med.* 2002;162:1401-1408.

2   Thaunat O, Beaumont C, Chatenoud L, et al. Anemia after late introduction of sirolimus may correlate with biochemical evidence of a chronic inflammatory state. *Transplantation.* 2005;80:1212-1219.

3   Pollock C, Johnson DW, Hörl WH, et al. Pure red cell aplasia induced by erythropoiesis-stimulating agents. *Clin J Am Soc Nephrol.* 2008;3:193-199.

4   López-Gómez JM, Pérez-Flores I, Jofré R, et al. Presence of a failed kidney transplant in patients who are on hemodialysis is associated with chronic inflammatory state and erythropoietin resistance. *J Am Soc Nephrol.* 2004;15:2494-2501.

Development of this book was supported by funding from Amgen

Chapter 5

Iron management

Iron deficiency: absolute versus functional

For the last two decades, iron deficiency has been categorized as either absolute or functional (see Table 2.2) [1].

Absolute iron deficiency implies that there is a deficiency in total body iron stores, such that there are inadequate levels of iron to supply the bone marrow. The two types of iron deficiency are often compared to a bank account. Absolute iron deficiency implies that there is simply not enough money in the bank to be able to make a withdrawal.

Functional iron deficiency is a condition in which there are normal or even increased levels of total body iron stores, but there is a failure to mobilize this iron for use by the bone marrow for erythropoiesis. To continue the bank account analogy, functional iron deficiency is illustrated by a condition in which there is an ample amount of money in a savings account, but it cannot be withdrawn on demand.

There are two types of functional iron deficiency. The first occurs when erythropoiesis is stimulated pharmacologically by ESA therapy. In this case, the demand for iron becomes so high that the iron supply becomes rate-limiting, and this is usually manifested by an increase in the percentage of hypochromic RBCs (Figure 5.1).

The second type of functional iron deficiency occurs when there is an inflammatory blockade of iron release from its stores in the reticulo-endothelial system. This is mediated by hepcidin, which is the master regulator of iron availability [2]. Hepcidin is upregulated in any acute

I. C. Macdougall, *Pocket Reference to Renal Anemia*,
DOI: 10.1007/978-1-907673-48-1_5, © Springer Healthcare 2013

Increase in hypochromic red blood cells following introduction of erythropoietin therapy

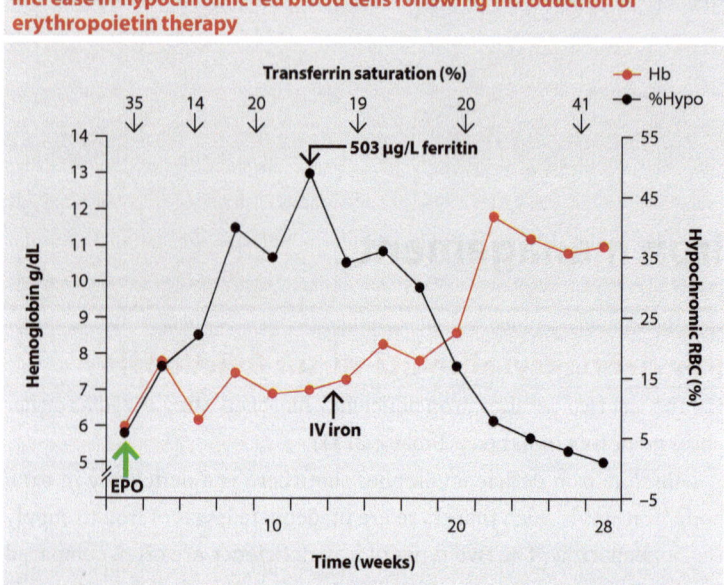

Figure 5.1 Increase in hypochromic red blood cells following introduction of erythropoietin therapy. RBC, red blood cell; EPO, erythropoietin; Hb, hemoglobin; Hypo, hypochromic.

or chronic inflammatory state, largely mediated via IL-6, although other proinflammatory cytokines may also play a part. Hepcidin exerts its physiological effect by binding to the cellular iron export protein, ferroportin, thereby shutting down any iron efflux from cells responsible for iron transport, such as duodenal enterocytes, macrophages, Kupffer cells, and splenocytes [2]. As one of the major rate-limiting steps in this process is the absorption of iron from the gut, it is possible to circumvent this by the administration of intravenous iron.

Detection of iron deficiency

There is no ideal test to confirm or refute the diagnosis of iron deficiency. The exception to this is a very low serum ferritin level (eg, <20 μg/L), which conclusively proves a diagnosis of absolute iron deficiency. There is no other cause for such a low serum ferritin level. However, the majority of patients have ferritin levels >20 μg/L, and yet many of them are also iron-deficient [1]. There are many other laboratory tests available for assessing iron status (Table 5.1). Serum iron on its own is unhelpful, but its relationship to the total iron binding capacity, expressed as a percentage (transferrin saturation), may support a diagnosis of iron insufficiency.

> *Learning point 11*
> A very low serum ferritin level (eg, <20 μg/L) conclusively proves a diagnosis of absolute iron deficiency, as there is no other cause for such a low level.

> *Learning point 12*
> Serum iron on its own is unhelpful as an indicator of iron deficiency, but its relationship to the total iron-binding capacity, expressed as a percentage (transferrin saturation), may be useful.

Markers of iron status

Marker	Characteristics
Serum ferritin	Reasonable marker of iron stores, but artificially elevated in the presence of inflammation or liver disease
Transferrin saturation	Subject to considerable diurnal variation; widely used in the US
Hypochromic red blood cells	Several studies suggest that this is the most sensitive/specific maker of iron deficiency, but needs to be performed on a fresh blood sample, and requires specific automated blood count analyzers, which are not widely available
Reticulocyte hemoglobin content	Also a fairly sensitive/specific maker of iron deficiency, but requires specific automated blood count analyzers, which are not widely available
MCV, MCH, MCHC	Abnormalities of these red blood cell indices will only occur in longstanding iron deficiency, and are therefore not a sensitive marker of iron status
Serum transferrin receptor	Used outside the nephrology setting, but not helpful in patients receiving ESA therapy, as this parameter will increase in either iron deficiency or enhanced erythropoiesis
Erythrocyte zinc protoporphyrin levels	Largely a research investigation with no practical applicability
Serum hepcidin levels	A novel biomarker of iron status, which remains experimental
Bone marrow	Useful investigation, but invasive and not practical for repeat assessments

Table 5.1 Markers of iron status. ESA, erythropoiesis-stimulating agent; MCV, mean corpuscular volume; MCH, mean cell hemoglobin; MCHC, mean corpuscular hemoglobin concentration.

Several studies have investigated the possible role of percentage hypochromic RBCs as an indicator of functional iron deficiency, and in a receptor operator curve analysis, this parameter was found to be the best in predicting a response to intravenous iron [3].

Serum transferrin receptor is useful in the diagnosis of iron deficiency outside the renal setting, but unfortunately for patients receiving erythropoietin therapy, it is less helpful, as the two drivers of an increase in serum transferrin receptor are iron deficiency and increased erythropoiesis [4]. Thus, for patients receiving ESA therapy this may be problematic. Erythrocyte zinc protoporphyrin remains a research investigation with no clinical applicability. Bone marrow examination for stainable iron may be helpful, but is clearly more invasive than other laboratory tests. As previously mentioned, the RBC indices such as MCH and MCHC may indicate a longstanding iron deficiency. Measurement of serum hepcidin is a novel biomarker, which has been investigated as a marker of iron insufficiency, but the results to date have been disappointing [5].

Iron supplementation: oral versus intravenous

Oral iron supplementation is simple and very cheap to administer. Unfortunately, in many patients with CKD, iron absorption is impaired due to hepcidin upregulation, and this renders oral iron supplementation ineffective [6].

Iron requirements in hemodialysis patients are too great for oral iron supplementation to keep pace with the demand, and this patient population is usually treated with intravenous iron. Nondialysis CKD patients, those on peritoneal dialysis, and kidney transplant recipients may receive oral iron first, although the other problem with this mode of administration is a high incidence of gastrointestinal side effects due to a local Fenton reaction at the site of the gastric or colonic mucosa [7]. Compliance with oral iron supplementation is often poor due to these side effects. Finally, iron absorption may be disrupted by many drugs, such as proton pump inhibitors (eg, omeprazole), phosphate binders, and certain antibiotics (eg, ciprofloxacin). Certain foods and tea may also impair dietary iron absorption [6].

If oral iron supplements are used, then the first choice is often ferrous sulphate. Attempts to reduce gastrointestinal side effects include taking iron supplements with meals, but this can also reduce their absorption. Other iron salts such as ferrous fumarate or ferrous succinate are sometimes reported as being better tolerated [6] because they contain lower amounts of elemental iron.

Intravenous iron is used widely in the CKD setting. Not only does this guarantee a readily available supply of iron, but it is extremely easy to administer to a hemodialysis population, who already have vascular access *in situ*. Thus, intravenous iron is usually administered on dialysis.

There are several intravenous iron preparations available worldwide (Table 5.2). The older iron preparations such as iron dextran carried a small but definite risk of anaphylaxis due to preformed dextran antibodies.

Requirements for a test dose and dosing schedule for various IV iron preparations licensed in the US and Europe, as per the product label

IV iron preparation	Country / region	Test dose required	Dosing schedule
Iron dextran – HMW (Dexferrum®)	US	Yes	100 mg bolus injection or slow IV infusion of up to 20 mg/kg
Iron dextran – LMW (INFeD®)	US	Yes	100 mg bolus injection or slow IV infusion of up to 20 mg/kg
Iron dextran – LMW (Cosmofer®)	Europe	Yes	100 mg bolus injection or slow IV infusion of up to 20 mg/kg
Iron sucrose (Venofer®)	US	No	100–200 mg bolus over 5–10 min
Iron sucrose (Venofer®)	Europe	Yes	100–200 mg bolus over 5–10 min
Ferric gluconate (Ferrlecit®)	US, Germany, Italy	No	62.5–12.5 mg bolus over 5–10 min
Ferumoxytol (Feraheme®)	US	No	510 mg bolus over 17 seconds
Ferumoxytol (Rienso®)	Europe	No	510 mg bolus over 17 seconds
Ferric carboxymaltose (Ferinject®)	Europe	No	500 mg bolus over 6 min / 1 g IV over 15 min (max 20 mg/kg)
Iron isomaltoside (Monofer®)	Europe	No	500 mg bolus over 30 min / 1 g IV over 60 min (max 20 mg/kg)

Table 5.2 Requirements for a test dose and dosing schedule for various IV iron preparations licensed in the US and Europe, as per the product label. HMW, high molecular weight; LMW, low molecular weight.

This has also been found to be more prevalent with high-molecular-weight iron dextran compared to low-molecular-weight iron dextran compounds [8].

Iron sucrose has been used for many years and is tried and tested in millions of doses worldwide. The usually administered dose is 100 mg or 200 mg, as tolerance at higher doses is reduced [9]. Iron gluconate is not licensed or marketed in the UK, but is used widely in the US, Italy, and Germany.

There are three new intravenous iron preparations recently licensed in Europe. These include ferric carboxymaltose (Ferinject®), iron isomaltoside (Monofer®), and ferumoxytol (Feraheme® in the US; Rienso® in Europe). These newer intravenous preparations may be administered in a larger dose over a shorter period of time, and do not require a test dose [10–12]. Animal studies suggest that there may be lower levels of free iron and oxidative stress with these newer preparations [13], although clinical and hard outcome data are lacking.

In some countries, such as France and Spain, iron sucrose "similars" are marketed. It is clear, however, that these products are very different from the iron sucrose originator (Venofer®) [14], with different levels of oxidative stress and also different efficacy [15]. At the present time, the iron sucrose similars are not available in the US or the UK.

The choice of intravenous iron preparation depends on the patient population to be treated. Thus, iron sucrose (Venofer) is often the intravenous iron of choice for hemodialysis patients (mainly due to cost), with boluses of 100 mg or 200 mg being administered once a month or once-weekly depending on iron requirements. Various sets of guidelines suggest that the optimum serum ferritin level for hemodialysis patients is 200–500 μg/L and the transferrin saturation level should be maintained above 20% [16]. If hypochromic RBCs can be measured, then this should be maintained below 10% [16].

For nondialysis patients, the choice of intravenous iron is a balance between patient convenience versus cost. Traditionally, many such patients received repeated boluses of intravenous iron sucrose, 200 mg at a time, but often three separate visits were needed to administer the required amount of intravenous iron. The newer intravenous iron preparations allow larger doses to be administered at a single visit, and thus doses of 500 mg or 1000 mg can be given as either a slow bolus injection or a fairly rapid intravenous infusion [10–12]. The newer intravenous irons, however, are slightly more costly, although this is balanced by savings on repeated outpatient visits and transport costs.

Reactions to intravenous iron

Over the years, intravenous iron administration has been notorious for causing immediate hypersensitivity-type anaphylactoid reactions. As previously mentioned, the iron dextran-containing preparation caused an IgE-mediated anaphylactic reaction, which resulted in several fatalities [17]. The modern-day intravenous iron preparations do not induce anaphylactic reactions, but may (not uncommonly) cause a hypotensive episode, characterized by sudden onset of dizziness and lightheadedness [18]. This can usually be managed by lying the patient supine without a need to give anti-allergic treatment such as adrenaline or steroids. The reaction is usually self-limiting after periods of a few minutes to up to a half hour. Admission to hospital is not usually necessary. These reactions to intravenous iron are rare but can be frightening for both the patient and the healthcare professional.

There is significant laboratory and animal evidence to suggest that intravenous iron may exacerbate acute bacterial infections, both by enhancing bacterial proliferation and by reducing neutrophil function, and for both these reasons, intravenous iron should not be given to patients with acute bacterial infection.

Learning point 13
IV iron should not be given to patients with acute bacterial infection.

References

1　Macdougall IC. Monitoring of iron status and iron supplementation in patients treated with erythropoietin. *Curr Opin Nephrol Hypertens*. 1994;3:620-625.

2　Babitt JL, Lin HY. Molecular mechanisms of hepcidin regulation: implications for the anemia of CKD. *Am J Kidney Dis*. 2010;55:726-741.

3   Tessitore N, Solero GP, Lippi G, et al. The role of iron status markers in predicting response to intravenous iron in haemodialysis patients on maintenance erythropoietin. *Nephrol Dial Transplant*. 2001;16:1416-1423.

4   Beguin Y. Soluble transferrin receptor for the evaluation of erythropoiesis and iron status. *Clin Chim Acta*. 2003;329:9-22.

5   Tessitore N, Girelli D, Campostrini N, et al. Hepcidin is not useful as a biomarker for iron needs in haemodialysis patients on maintenance erythropoiesis-stimulating agents. *Nephrol Dial Transplant*. 2010;25:3996-4002.

6   Macdougall IC. Strategies for iron supplementation: oral versus intravenous. *Kidney Int Suppl*. 1999;69:S61-S66.

7   Charytan C, Qunibi W, Bailie GR; Venofer Clinical Studies Group. Comparison of intravenous iron sucrose to oral iron in the treatment of anemic patients with chronic kidney disease not on dialysis. *Nephron Clin Pract*. 2005;100:c55-c62.

8   Bailie GR, Hörl WH, Verhoef JJ. Differences in spontaneously reported hypersensitivity and serious adverse events for intravenous iron preparations: comparison of Europe and North America. *Arzneimittelforschung*. 2011;61:267-275.

9   Chandler G, Harchowal J, Macdougall IC. Intravenous iron sucrose: establishing a safe dose. *Am J Kidney Dis*. 2001;38:988-991.

10   Ferinject [package insert]. Neuilly-sur-Seine, France: Vifor Pharma; 2011.

11   Monofer [package insert]. Holbaek, Denmark: Pharmacosmos; 2009.

12   Feraheme [package insert]. Lexington, MA: AMAG Pharmaceuticals; 2011.

13   Toblli JE, Cao G, Oliveri L, Angerosa M. Assessment of the extent of oxidative stress induced by intravenous ferumoxytol, ferric carboxymaltose, iron sucrose and iron dextran in a nonclinical model. *Arzneimittelforschung*. 2011;61:399-410.

14   Venofer [package insert]. Shirley, NY: American Regent; 2011.

15   Toblli JE, Cao G, Oliveri L, Angerosa M. Comparison of oxidative stress and inflammation induced by different intravenous iron sucrose similar preparations in a rat model. *Inflamm Allergy Drug Targets*. 2012;11:66-78.

16   Locatelli F, Aljama P, Barany P, et al. Revised European best practice guidelines for the management of anaemia in patients with chronic renal failure. *Nephrol Dial Transplant*. 2004;19(suppl 2):ii1-47.

17   Bailie GR, Clark JA, Lane CE, et al. Hypersensitivity reactions and deaths associated with intravenous iron preparations. *Nephrol Dial Transplant*. 2005;20:1443-1449.

18   National Kidney Foundation. KDIGO clinical practice guideline for anemia in chronic kidney disease. *Kidney Int Suppl*. 2012;2:v-335.

Development of this book was supported by funding from Amgen

Chapter 6

Erythropoiesis-stimulating agent therapy

Erythropoiesis-stimulating agents remain the cornerstone of CKD anemia management. They were introduced in 1990 and transformed the management of anemia in dialysis patients, many of whom were transfusion-dependent and iron overloaded.

Epoetins (including "biosimilars")

The first generation of ESAs were the recombinant human erythropoietins, epoetin alfa (Epogen®, Eprex®) and epoetin beta (NeoRecormon®). Both products are fairly short-acting, with a plasma half-life of between 6 and 8 hours, and this requires them to be administered by intravenous or subcutaneous injection two or three times weekly [1]. Following the expiration of the patent for these products, several biosimilar epoetins have recently appeared on the market, including epoetin zeta (Retacrit®, Silapo®) and biosimilar epoetin alfa (Binocrit®, Hexal®, Abseamed®) [2,3]. Another recombinant human erythropoietin (epoetin theta; Eporatio®) has also recently been licensed [4].

These products, which have been approved by the European Medicines Agency, have been shown to be *bioequivalent* to an "originator" epoetin, both in terms of efficacy and safety within prespecified limits, but are not *identical* to the originator. With such a complex molecule, it is impossible to replicate exactly the original biochemical structure of the originator, as can be easily achieved for small molecule "generic" products. In addition, there are hundreds of "copy" epoetins around the world that have

I. C. Macdougall, *Pocket Reference to Renal Anemia*,
DOI: 10.1007/978-1-907673-48-1_6, © Springer Healthcare 2013

not been approved through the European Medicine Agency biosimilar regulatory process, and may therefore differ considerably in physico-chemical properties, efficacy, and safety from the originator epoetins [5].

Darbepoetin alfa

The main difference between darbepoetin alfa (Aranesp®) and the epoet-ins is the presence of an additional two N-linked carbohydrate chains to enhance the metabolic stability of the molecule in vivo (Figure 6.1). Thus, the intravenous half-life of darbepoetin alfa is approximately 25 hours, while the subcutaneous half-life is between 48 and 70 hours. This property allows less frequent dosing, and this product is effective once-weekly or once every 2 weeks. It may also be administered subcutaneously once-monthly for maintaining the Hb target in nondialysis patients [6].

Darbepoetin alfa: a molecule with two more N-linked glycosylation chains than recombinant human erythropoietin

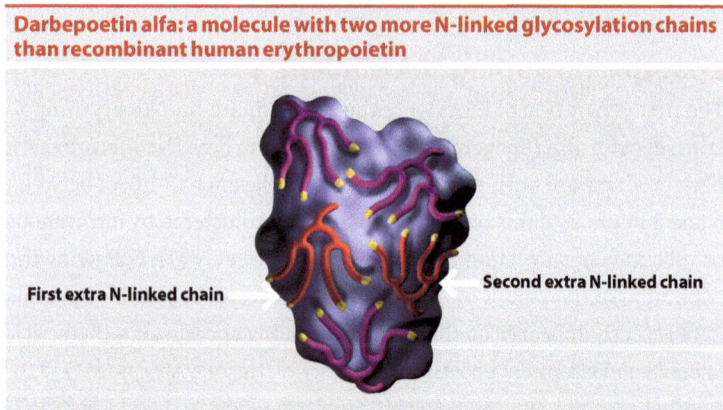

First extra N-linked chain

Second extra N-linked chain

Figure 6.1 Darbepoetin alfa: a molecule with two more N-linked glycosylation chains than recombinant human erythropoietin. Five amino acids on the recombinant human erythropoietin polypeptide backbone were changed to introduce two new N-linked carbohydrate recognition sites, resulting in darbepoetin alfa. It is approximately 51% carbohydrate by weight, and its two extra carbohydrate side chains attach precisely in the region where the amino acid sequence has been altered.

Methoxypolyethylene glycol epoetin beta

Methoxypolyethylene glycol epoetin beta (Continuous Erythropoietin Receptor Activator [C.E.R.A]; Mircera®) was created by attaching a pegyla-tion chain to the epoetin beta molecule (Figure 6.2). This considerably prolonged the circulating half-life of the molecule to around 130 hours, which allows for once-monthly administration [7]. This is particularly useful in nondialysis patients.

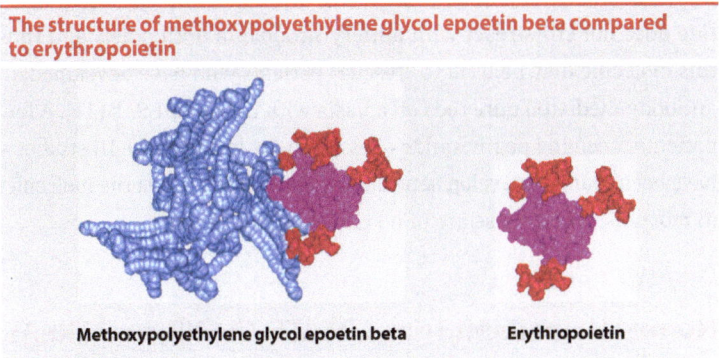

Figure 6.2 The structure of methoxypolyethylene glycol epoetin beta compared to erythropoietin. Blue: methoxypolyethylene glycol epoetin beta; purple: erythropoietin; red: N-linked glycosylation chains.

Peginesatide

In March 2012, peginesatide was licensed as an ESA in the US (Omontys®) for dialysis patients. Peginesatide is an erythropoietin-mimetic peptide that has no structural homology with erythropoietin, but shares the same biological and functional properties as the native or recombinant protein. Thus, it simulates erythropoiesis by binding to the erythropoietin receptor and evoking the same intracellular signaling cascade (Figure 6.3) [8].

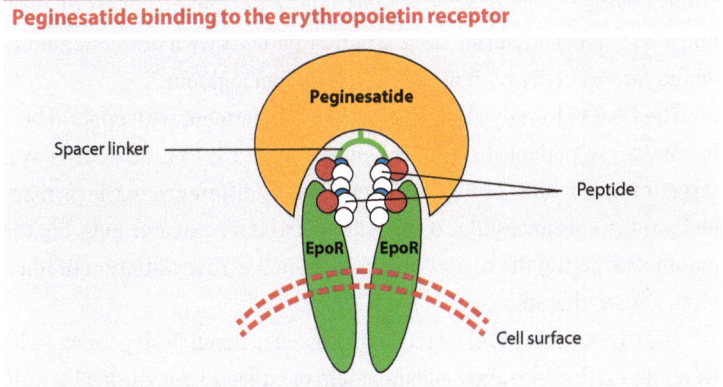

Figure 6.3 Peginesatide binding to the erythropoietin receptor. EpoR, erythropoietin receptor.

Four large Phase III clinical trials of this product were conducted (PEARL 1 & 2; EMERALD 1 & 2), allowing a cumulative exposure in approximately 2600 patients [9,10]. In contrast to the other licensed ESAs, peginesatide does not cross-react with antierythropoietin antibodies, and thus this molecule may be used to "rescue" patients who have developed an antibody-mediated pure red cell aplasia with the other ESAs [11]. A few patients receiving peginesatide – less than 1% in the Phase III studies – have been found to develop neutralizing antibodies against the molecule; in most instances, these are of no clinical significance.

Normal Hematocrit Trial, CREATE, CHOIR, and TREAT

Four large randomized controlled trials (US Normal Hematocrit Trial [12], CREATE [13], CHOIR [14], and TREAT [15]) all suggested potential safety concerns with the use of ESA therapy to normalize the hemoglobin concentration.

The **Normal Hematocrit Trial** [12], conducted in 1233 US hemodialysis patients treated with epoetin alfa, was the first to be published. This study was stopped prematurely, as the group of patients randomized to a target hemoglobin of 14 g/dL had a higher incidence of vascular access thrombosis, and a borderline statistically significant higher incidence of the primary composite endpoint (death or first non-fatal myocardial infarction). To be eligible for this trial, however, patients had to have clinical evidence of congestive heart failure or ischemic heart disease, and it was not clear at this stage whether patients with less comorbidity would fare as badly with normalization of hemoglobin.

The **CREATE** study [13] then compared treatment with epoetin beta in nondialysis patients to a target hemoglobin of 13–15 g/dL with a lower target range of 10.5–11.5 g/dL. There was no difference in the primary endpoint (a cardiovascular composite) between the two groups, but the patients targeting the higher hemoglobin had earlier initiation of renal replacement therapy.

The **CHOIR** study [14] was also conducted in nondialysis patients, who were randomized to target a hemoglobin of either 13.5 g/dL or 11.3 g/dL with epoetin alfa therapy. The primary endpoint was a composite of death, myocardial infarction, stroke, or hospitalization for heart failure, and the group of patients targeting the higher hemoglobin experienced a greater number of events (125 vs 97; P=0.03).

This was followed by even more definitive conclusions from the **TREAT** study [15], which was a randomized double-blind, placebo-controlled trial in 4038 nondialysis diabetic CKD patients, half of whom were randomized to target a hemoglobin of 13 g/dL with darbepoetin alfa, while the other half received placebo (being rescued only if their hemoglobin fell below 9 g/dL). Targeting the higher hemoglobin concentration showed a significant reduction in the use of blood transfusions, but only a fairly modest improvement in quality of life. Also, TREAT failed to show a reduction in time to death or a cardiovascular event (eg, myocardial infarction, congestive heart failure, or stroke) or end-stage renal disease. Also, the risk of venous and arterial thromboembolism increased significantly, and the risk of stroke was nearly double in patients in the higher hemoglobin arm (101 patients [5.0%] vs 53 patients [2.6%]; hazard ratio 1.9; 95% confidence interval, 1.4–2.7; Figure 6.4).

Furthermore, although there was no significant difference in the overall number of patients reporting a cancer-related adverse event (6.9% in the darbepoetin alfa group and 6.4% in the placebo group (P=0.53),

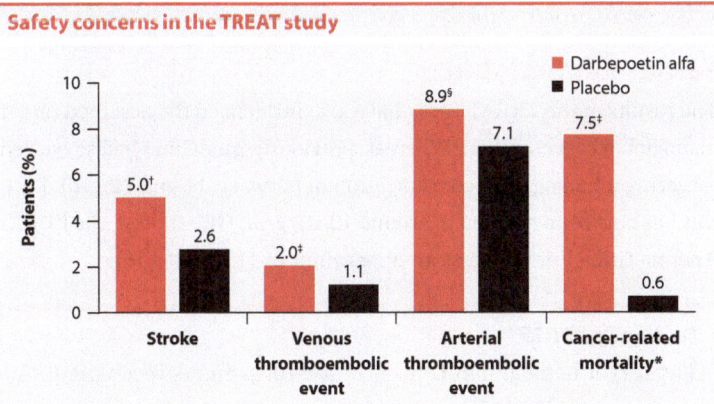

Figure 6.4 Safety concerns in the TREAT study. *Among patients with a history of malignancy at baseline; †P<0.001 versus placebo; ‡P=0.02 versus placebo; §P=0.04 versus placebo. TREAT, Trial to Reduce cardiovascular Events with Aranesp Therapy. Based on data from Pfeffer et al [15].

among the subgroup of patients who had a history of malignancy at baseline, there was a greater than tenfold increase in cancer-related death in the higher hemoglobin arm compared to the placebo arm (7.5% compared with 0.6%; P=0.002; Figure 6.4).

Trigger hemoglobin concentration

The results from the TREAT study indicated that, in contrast to what was previously believed, many patients with CKD randomized to the placebo group could manage for significant periods of time without active ESA therapy. This strongly influenced the the recently published Kidney Disease: Improving Global Outcomes (KDIGO) 2012 Anemia Guideline, in which it was suggested that ESA therapy should be introduced somewhere around 9 or 10 g/dL, with the aim of preventing the hemoglobin level from falling below 9 g/dL [16]. This trigger hemoglobin concentration is somewhat lower than was previously recommended in both US and European clinical practice guidelines.

> *Learning point 14*
> The trigger hemoglobin concentration for initiating ESA therapy should be somewhere around 9 or 10 g/dL, with the aim of preventing patients' hemogolobin levels from falling below 9 g/dL [16].

Target hemoglobin

The results of the TREAT study have also influenced the accepted target hemoglobin concentration. Whereas, previously, guidelines had suggested targeting a hemoglobin concentration of between 11 and 12 g/dL [17], this has now been reduced to around 10–12 g/dL [18]. Indeed, the KDIGO Anemia Guideline suggests an upper limit of 11.5 g/dL [16].

> *Learning point 15*
> The target hemoglobin concentration for patients receiving ESA therapy should be individualized, but should be somewhere around 10–12 g/dL [18].

Erythropoiesis-stimulating agent therapy and the risk of malignancy

Background and rationale for concerns regarding the safety of ESA therapy in patients with known or suspected malignancy: what we know and what we do not know

The latest KDIGO Anemia Guideline [16] expresses a concern that was not highlighted in previous international guidelines regarding the safety of ESA therapy in patients with known or suspected malignancy. This increased concern arose following the latest evidence review conducted specifically for the KDIGO Anemia Guideline, and was strongly influenced by some of the findings from the TREAT study reported in November 2009 [15].

Safety concerns regarding malignancy from the TREAT study

No patient with active or suspected malignancy was allowed to be recruited to the TREAT study – this was one of the exclusion criteria. However, patients with a previous malignancy from at least 5 years ago, and who were deemed to be cured, could be included in the study.

In this latter subgroup of patients, an analysis of the rate of cancer-related mortality was conducted, and there was a more than tenfold increase in this compared with the placebo group. Given that this was not the primary objective of the study, this result needs to be interpreted with caution; however, the magnitude of this effect is hard to ignore. The explanation for this result is also not clear, despite further post-hoc analyses.

Another finding from the TREAT study was a doubling of the incidence of venous thromboembolism in patients receiving ESA therapy compared to those receiving placebo. It is well-recognized that patients with cancer are predisposed to venous thromboembolism, and indeed there is strong evidence from the oncology literature that ESA therapy can exacerbate this risk [19]. Although the doses of ESA therapy used in the oncology setting are several orders of magnitude greater than those used in the CKD setting, there remains a concern that ESA therapy can worsen the risk of venous thromboembolism, possibly via an effect on platelet function, and for this reason, caution is recommended.

Can ESA therapy exacerbate the growth of a malignant cell clone?

There is much controversy over whether or not ESA therapy, as a growth factor, can exacerbate the growth of a malignant cell clone. One of the earliest oncology trials of erythropoietin therapy for anemia associated with head and neck cancer suggested that patients whose tumor tissue screened positive for the erythropoietin receptor had a worse survival than those who were negative for the erythropoietin receptor [20]. This was one of the earliest pieces of evidence to relate ESA therapy to worsened cancer-related survival.

This work has since been discredited: it is now clear that the antibody used for detecting the erythropoietin receptor cross-reacts with heat shock protein, and that tumor tissue positive for heat shock protein indicates a worse prognosis. Thus the link between ESA therapy and the erythropoietin receptor positivity was flawed.

Many studies have since been conducted on whether certain cancers or cancer cell lines have a functional erythropoietin receptor [21–24]. The methodology used for detecting the erythropoietin receptor has been less than robust, and this has led to misleading results. Recently, Elliott and colleagues have produced a monoclonal antibody against the erythropoietin receptor, which is believed to be of better quality than that used in previous studies [21]. Several studies now suggest that the erythropoietin receptor is not as ubiquitous as was once believed, and even if anatomically present on the cell surface, there is still uncertainty as to whether it is truly functional [21–24].

Thus, the recent laboratory data have cast some doubt as to the role of erythropoietin in exacerbating malignancy. Until there is further clarification on this issue, however, caution is still advised in any patient with a known or suspected malignancy.

Erythropoiesis-stimulating agent therapy and the risk of stroke

The latest KDIGO Anemia Guideline [16] expresses a concern that was not highlighted in previous international guidelines regarding the use of ESA therapy in patients with a previous stroke, or at a high risk of having a stroke. This concern arose following the latest evidence review conducted specifically for the KDIGO Anemia Guideline, and was strongly influenced by some of the findings from the TREAT study reported in November 2009 [15].

Safety concerns regarding stroke from the TREAT study

One of the secondary endpoints in the TREAT study, which was a component of the primary composite endpoint, was the development of stroke during the trial. Overall, 154 of the 4038 patients recruited to the study had a stroke: 101/2012 (5.0%) in the darbepoetin alfa arm and 53/2026 (2.6%) in the placebo arm (hazard ratio 1.9; 95% confidence interval, 1.4–2.7). Thus, in short, there was a doubling of the risk of stroke in patients randomized to the active ESA arm compared with placebo.

Was this finding unprecedented?

Almost, but not completely. An earlier randomized controlled trial in early hemodialysis patients had also shown a higher event rate in patients randomized to hemoglobin normalization versus partial correction of anemia [25]. However, the event rate in this study was very low – only 12 patients having a stroke in the hemoglobin normalization arm and 4 having a stroke in the partial correction of anemia arm (P=0.045).

Further analysis of the TREAT study findings

The data from the TREAT study were subjected to a further detailed analysis to see if any baseline variables could account for the development of stroke in this study population [26]. A multivariate logistic regression model was used to identify baseline predictors of stroke. A number of other factors, including post-randomization blood pressure, hemoglobin level, platelet count, or treatment dose were also assessed using a nested case–control analysis (1:10 matching) identifying nonstroke controls with propensity matching to see if any of these factors could account for the increased risk related to darbepoetin alfa. None of the baseline variables nor any of the factors in the case–control analysis could be used to mitigate the risk of darbepoetin alfa-related stroke. Although the absolute risk of stroke was greater if there was a history of previous stroke, the relative risk of stroke in patients treated with darbepoetin alfa remained at 2 to 1 versus placebo [26].

Is there a biological rationale for the potential of ESA therapy to exacerbate stroke?

Exacerbation of cardiovascular adverse events may be mediated via the pleiotropic effects of erythropoietic agents – more specifically, their effect on endothelin and platelet function – and this has been nicely reviewed by Vaziri and Zhou [27].

Implications for anemia management

Physicians using ESAs should be aware of the potential for exacerbating stroke, and in any patients believed to be high risk, the benefits versus risks of using ESA therapy should be weighed up carefully. If ESA therapy is used, target hemoglobin concentrations should not exceed 11.5 or 12 g/dL in order to reduce the risk of this potentially devastating adverse effect.

Poor response to erythropoiesis-stimulating agent therapy

There are two types of poor response to ESAs. The first is a failure to show an increase in hemoglobin concentration despite repeated increases in ESA dose. The second is characterized by a loss of response to treatment, again despite increased ESA doses. Both of these conditions require a careful systematic approach.

The causes of hyporesponsiveness to ESA therapy are several (Table 6.1). Investigating a patient who is showing hyporesponsiveness to ESA therapy merits a step-wise approach (Figure 6.5). If the patient is self-injecting, compliance with therapy should be questioned and confirmed. The reticulocyte count may give a clue as to whether there is a primary problem with erythropoiesis, or whether the bone marrow is already working overtime but the RBC survival is reduced as a result of bleeding or hemolysis.

The possibility of either absolute or functional iron deficiency should be entertained, and a trial of intravenous iron may be helpful. A raised

Causes of hyporesponsiveness to erythropoiesis-stimulating agent therapy	
Common	**Less common**
Iron deficiency	Blood loss
Infection/inflammation	Hyperparathyroidism
Underdialysis	Aluminum toxicity
	Vitamin B_{12}/folate deficiency
	Hemolysis
	Bone marrow disorders
	Hemoglobinopathies
	Angiotensin-converting enzyme inhibitors
	Carnitine deficiency
	Obesity (in subcutaneous administration)
	Anti-EPO antibodies (pure red cell aplasia)

Table 6.1 Causes of hyporesponsiveness to erythropoiesis-stimulating agent therapy.
EPO, erythropoietin.

C-reactive protein may suggest active infection or inflammation, and this should be vigorously investigated. Occult conditions such as tuberculosis or malignancy may prove somewhat elusive. An increase in dialysis prescription, and/or a change from conventional hemodialysis to hemodiafiltration may be of benefit. Screening for vitamin B_{12} or folate deficiency, blood loss, or hemolysis may be indicated. A sharp fall in hemoglobin coupled with a very low reticulocyte count should alert the physician to the very rare condition of antibody-mediated pure red cell aplasia. Bone marrow examination may be required to exclude some hematological conditions such as myelodysplastic syndrome. A higher reticulocyte count makes it more likely that bleeding or hemolysis is the cause, and a full hemolytic screen and possible gastrointestinal investigations may be indicated.

> *Learning point 16*
> In patients showing a suboptimal response to ESA therapy, the reticulocyte count may provide helpful information. If low, then erythropoiesis is probably suppressed or deficient, whereas a high reticulocyte count might suggest bleeding or hemolysis.

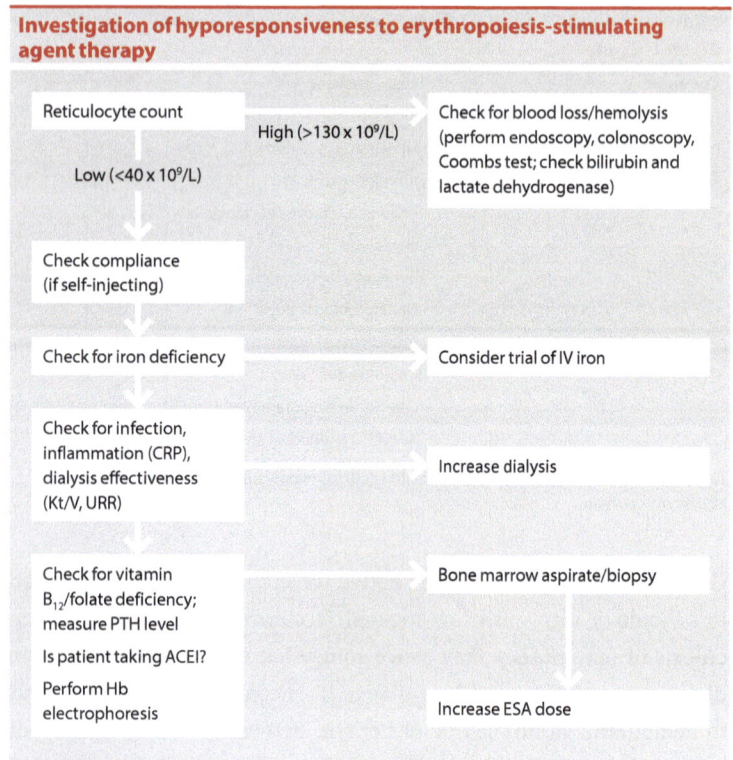

Figure 6.5 Investigation of hyporesponsiveness to erythropoiesis-stimulating agent therapy. ACEI, angiotensin-converting enzyme inhibitors; CRP, C-reactive protein; ESA, erythropoiesis-stimulating agent; Hb, hemoglobin; PTH, parathyroid hormone; URR, urea reduction ratio.

Whereas previously physicians tended to escalate the dose of ESA therapy to higher levels, recent randomized controlled trials have suggested possible harm in using high doses in erythropoietin-resistant patients [12–15]. It is not clear whether the poor outcomes in this situation are due to the high doses of ESA therapy per se, or whether this simply represents a group of patients who are generally more ill. Nevertheless, repeated dose escalation is no longer advised, and a maximum dose of epoetin of around 15,000 units per week in divided doses seems reasonable. This translates into a weekly dose of approximately 75 µg of darbepoetin alfa, or a monthly dose of approximately 300 µg of methoxypolyethylene glycol epoetin beta.

Adjuvant therapy

Since the earliest days of ESA use, it became clear that intravenous iron supplementation enhanced the response to erythropoietin therapy, and allowed lower doses to be used. It became rapidly apparent that an inadequate iron supply to the bone marrow was a rate-limiting step in the process of erythropoiesis.

Over the years, several other adjuvant therapies have been studied to ascertain whether similar results could be seen with these agents [28–34]. The studies included trials of vitamin C, D, and E supplementation, as well as vitamin B_{12} and folate supplementation, L-carnitine supplements, androgens, and pentoxifylline. Some of these studies were conducted in a placebo-controlled, double-blind fashion (eg, carnitine [28]), but the cohorts in all studies were small, and the studies have not been of a high enough caliber to influence clinical practice guidelines or support the use of any of these adjuvants in the routine management of renal anemia.

Nevertheless, there may be individual instances when these adjuvants could be considered. Certainly, if there is evidence of vitamin B_{12} or folate insufficiency in any patient, then the deficient vitamin should be supplemented. The vitamin C (ascorbic acid) studies were conducted in patients with relative iron overload, and the rationale for the use of this therapy was that it may mobilize iron from its body stores [29]. Pentoxifylline (oxpentifylline) was studied in an open-label fashion in a very small number of patients with chronic inflammation [34], and although positive results were seen, again this cannot support routine use of this treatment. A larger randomized placebo-controlled trial is, however, currently being conducted in Australia [35], and the results are awaited with interest.

In short, the use of adjuvant therapy beyond intravenous iron does not have a strong evidence-base, but can be considered in an individual patient.

References

1 Halstenson CE, Macres M, Katz SA, et al. Comparative pharmacokinetics and pharmacodynamics of epoetin alfa and epoetin beta. *Clin Pharmacol Ther*. 1991;50:702-712.
2 Retacrit [package insert]. Warwickshire, UK: Hospira; 2010.
3 Binocrit [package insert]. Kundl, Austria: Sandoz; 2010.
4 Eporatio [package insert]. Ulm, Germany: Merckle Biotec; 2009.

5   Macdougall IC, Ashenden M. Current and upcoming erythropoiesis-stimulating agents, iron products, and other novel anemia medications. *Adv Chronic Kidney Dis*. 2009;16:117-130.

6   Aranesp [package insert]. Thousand Oaks, CA: Amgen; 2012.

7   Mircera [package insert]. Welwyn Garden City, UK: Hoffmann-La Roche; 2007.

8   Fan Q, Leuther KK, Holmes CP, et al. Preclinical evaluation of Hematide, a novel erythropoiesis stimulating agent, for the treatment of anemia. *Exp Hematol*. 2006;34:1303-1311.

9   Macdougall IC, Provenzano R, Sharma A, et al. Peginesatide for anemia in patients with chronic kidney disease not receiving dialysis. *N Engl J Med*. 2013;368:320-332.

10 Fishbane S, Schiller B, Locatelli F, et al. Peginesatide in patients with anemia undergoing hemodialysis. *N Engl J Med*. 2013;368:307-319.

11 Macdougall IC, Rossert J, Casadevall N, et al. A peptide-based erythropoietin-receptor agonist for pure red-cell aplasia. *N Engl J Med*. 2009;361:1848-1855.

12 Besarab A, Bolton WK, Browne JK, et al. The effects of normal as compared with low hematocrit values in patients with cardiac disease who are receiving hemodialysis and epoetin. *N Engl J Med*. 1998;339:584-590.

13 Drueke TB, Locatelli F, Clyne N, et al. Normalization of hemoglobin level in patients with chronic kidney disease and anemia. *N Engl J Med*. 2006;355:2071-2084.

14 Singh AK, Szczech L, Tang KL, et al. Correction of anemia with epoetin alfa in chronic kidney disease. *N Engl J Med*. 2006;355:2085-2098.

15 Pfeffer MA, Burdmann EA, Chen C-Y, et al. A trial of darbepoetin alfa in type 2 diabetes and chronic kidney disease. *N Engl J Med*. 2009;361:2019-2032.

16 National Kidney Foundation. KDIGO clinical practice guideline for anemia in chronic kidney disease. *Kidney Int Suppl*. 2012;2:v-335.

17 National Kidney Foundation. KDOQI clinical practice guideline and clinical practice recommendations for anemia in chronic kidney disease: 2007 update of hemoglobin target. *Am J Kidney Dis*. 2007;50:471-530.

18 National Institute for Health and Clinical Excellence. Anaemia management in people with chronic kidney disease. http://guidance.nice.org.uk/CG114. Updated November 2012. Accessed February 6, 2013.

19 Bennett CL, Silver SM, Djulbegovic B, et al. Venous thromboembolism and mortality associated with recombinant erythropoietin and darbepoetin administration for the treatment of cancer-associated anemia. *JAMA*. 2008;299:914-924.

20 Henke M, Laszig R, Rübe C, et al. Erythropoietin to treat head and neck cancer patients with anaemia undergoing radiotherapy: randomised, double-blind, placebo-controlled trial. *Lancet*. 2003;362:1255-1260.

21 Elliott S, Busse L, Bass MB, et al. Anti-Epo receptor antibodies do not predict Epo receptor expression. *Blood*. 2006;107:1892-1895.

22 Fandrey J. Erythropoietin receptors on tumor cells: what do they mean? *Oncologist*. 2008;13(suppl 3):16-20.

23 Swift S, Ellison AR, Kassner P, et al. Absence of functional EpoR expression in human tumor cell lines. *Blood*. 2010;115:4254-4263.

24 Sinclair AM, Coxon A, McCaffery I, et al. Functional erythropoietin receptor is undetectable in endothelial, cardiac, neuronal, and renal cells. *Blood*. 2010;115:4264-4272.

25 Parfrey PS, Foley RN, Wittreich BH, Sullivan DJ, Zagari MJ, Frei D. Double-blind comparison of full and partial anemia correction in incident hemodialysis patients without symptomatic heart disease. *J Am Soc Nephrol*. 2005;16:2180-2189.

26 Skali H, Parving HH, Parfrey PS, et al. Stroke in patients with type 2 diabetes mellitus, chronic kidney disease, and anemia treated with darbepoetin alfa: the trial to reduce cardiovascular events with Aranesp therapy (TREAT) experience. *Circulation*. 2011;124:2903-2908.

27 Vaziri ND, Zhou XJ. Potential mechanisms of adverse outcomes in trials of anemia correction with erythropoietin in chronic kidney disease. *Nephrol Dial Transplant*. 2009;24:1082-1088.

28 Labonia WD. L-Carnitine effects on anemia in hemodialyzed patients treated with erythropoietin. *Am J Kidney Dis*. 1995;26:757-764.

29 Tarng DC, Huang TP. A parallel, comparative study of intravenous iron versus intravenous ascorbic acid for erythropoietin-hyporesponsive anaemia in haemodialysis patients with iron overload. *Nephrol Dial Transplant*. 1998;13:2867-2872.

30 Albitar S, Genin R, Fen-Chong M, et al. High-dose alfacalcidol improves anaemia in patients on haemodialysis. *Nephrol Dial Transplant*. 1997;12:514-518.

31 Ballal SH, Domoto DT, Polack DC, et al. Androgens potentiate the effects of erythropoietin in the treatment of anemia of end-stage renal disease. *Am J Kidney Dis*. 1991;17:29-33.

32 Pronai W, Riegler-Keil M, Silberbauer K, Stockenhuber F. Folic acid supplementation improves erythropoietin response. *Nephron*. 1995;71:395-400.

33 Brox AG, Zhang F, Guyda H, Gagnon RF. Subtherapeutic erythropoietin and insulin-like growth factor-1 correct the anemia of chronic renal failure in the mouse. *Kidney Int*. 1996;50:937-943.

34 Cooper A, Mikhail A, Lethbridge MW, Kemeny DM, Macdougall IC. Pentoxifylline improves hemoglobin levels in patients with erythropoietin-resistant anemia in renal failure. *J Am Soc Nephrol*. 2004;15:1877-1882.

35 Johnson DW, Hawley CM, Rosser B, et al. Oxpentifylline versus placebo in the treatment of erythropoietin-resistant anaemia: a randomized controlled trial. *BMC Nephrol*. 2008;9:8.

Development of this book was supported by funding from Amgen

Chapter 7

Blood transfusions

Prior to 1990, RBC transfusions were very frequently used in chronic hemodialysis patients. The advent of erythropoietin therapy led to a dramatic reduction in the incidence of transfusions: the Annual Report of the US Renal Data System in 2009 indicated a halving of blood transfusions from approximately 14% to approximately 7% over the first decade of ESA use (Figure 7.1) [1].

Reduction in blood transfusions following the introduction of erythropoietin as a therapeutic agent

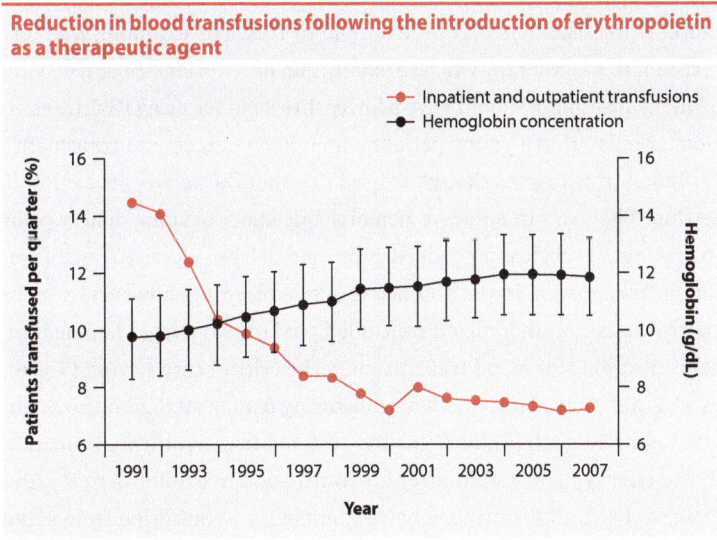

Figure 7.1 Reduction in blood transfusions following the introduction of erythropoietin as a therapeutic agent.

I. C. Macdougall, *Pocket Reference to Renal Anemia*,
DOI: 10.1007/978-1-907673-48-1_7, © Springer Healthcare 2013

Given the safety concerns associated with ESA therapy, however, it is likely that the use of RBC transfusions will once again increase. The major concerns associated with blood transfusion use are the fairly rare occurrence of transmission of infectious agents and some rare but life-threatening transfusion reactions, such as transfusion-related lung injury and transfusion-related acute circulatory overload. However, the main concern with blood transfusion use in patients with CKD is the risk of human leukocyte antigen sensitization [2]. Recent data from the US Renal Data System confirm that this remains a problem, and human leukocyte antigen sensitization is associated with a longer waiting time for kidney transplantation, reduced likelihood of receiving a kidney transplant, and poor graft outcomes if transplanted [1]. Thus, every attempt should be made to avoid blood transfusions where possible, particularly in younger patients.

The current focus in renal anemia management is individualization of treatment [3], and the balance between the use of ESA therapy versus blood transfusions is a good example of this. For example, patients resistant to ESA therapy who are elderly and have no chance of receiving a kidney transplant should have a lower threshold for using RBC transfusions compared to a young patient who is keen to receive a transplant.

Blood transfusions should be used in either the acute or the chronic setting. Their use in an acute hemorrhagic state, or immediately prior to any urgent surgical procedure, is beyond debate. Elective transfusion for chronic anemia in the absence of active bleeding, however, is more controversial. A randomized controlled trial of two trigger hemoglobin concentrations for blood transfusion in the critical care setting (7 g/dL vs 10 g/dL) showed no benefit in transfusing patients if their hemoglobin was below 10 g/dL [4], and this has resulted in a significant reduction in the trigger hemoglobin level for transfusion to around 7 to 8 g/dL. Even in the cardiac setting, when patients may be suffering from acute coronary syndrome, the use of blood transfusion above a hemoglobin level of 8 g/dL has been critically questioned [5]. Thus, in the absence of acute bleeding, there is little indication to transfuse a patient above 7 or 8 g/dL unless a surgical procedure is planned in which significant blood loss might be expected [3].

Learning point 17

In the absence of acute bleeding, there is little indication to transfuse a patient with hemoglobin levels above 7 or 8 g/dL unless a surgical procedure is planned in which significant blood loss might be expected [3].

References

1 US Renal Data System. *USRDS 2009 Annual Data Report: Atlas of Chronic Kidney Disease and End-Stage Renal Disease in the United States*. Bethesda, MD: National Institutes of Health, National Institute of Diabetes and Digestive and Kidney Diseases; 2009.

2 Obrador GT, Macdougall IC. Impact of red cell transfusions on future kidney transplantation. *Clin J Am Soc Nephrol*. 2012 Oct 18. [Epub ahead of print].

3 National Kidney Foundation. KDIGO clinical practice guideline for anemia in chronic kidney disease. *Kidney Int Suppl*. 2012;2:v-335.

4 Hebert PC, Wells G, Blajchman MA, et al. A multicenter, randomized, controlled clinical trial of transfusion requirements in critical care. Transfusion Requirements in Critical Care Investigators, Canadian Critical Care Trials Group. *N Engl J Med*. 1999; 340: 409-41.

5 Kansagara D, Dyer EAW, Englander H, Freeman M, Kagen D. Treatment of anemia in patients with heart disease: a systematic review. The National Center for Biotechnology Information website. www.ncbi.nlm.nih.gov/books/NBK83423/pdf/TOC.pdf. Accessed February 6, 2013.

Development of this book was supported by funding from Amgen

Chapter 8

Guidelines on the management of renal anemia

Ever since ESA therapy was introduced, clinical practice guidelines on the management of anemia in patients with CKD have been devised in various parts of the world. Thus, US, European, UK (National Institute for Health and Clinical Excellence [NICE]), Australian, Canadian, and Japanese anemia guidelines have all been published over the last two decades (Table 8.1). The guidelines have discussed most of the issues outlined in this chapter, focusing mainly on ESA and iron management, and there has been an evolution of recommendations over time. Since 2010, the Work Group of the KDIGO Anemia Guideline has reviewed the latest evidence on the management of anemia in CKD patients, and their final report was published in August 2012. This is a comprehensive review of the latest literature, but the main points are summarized in Table 8.2. Prior to the KDIGO Anemia Guideline publication, the European Renal Best Practice Group published a report of their latest recommendations (Table 8.3). Finally, following publication of the TREAT study, the UK NICE Group revised their anemia guideline with regard to trigger and target hemoglobin only. No review of iron management was conducted for this update, but the main features of the NICE Anemia Guideline (published in February 2011) were a trigger hemoglobin concentration of 11 g/dL for the use of ESA therapy, and a target ("aspirational") hemoglobin range of 10–12 g/dL.

I. C. Macdougall, *Pocket Reference to Renal Anemia*,
DOI: 10.1007/978-1-907673-48-1_8, © Springer Healthcare 2013

Clinical Practice Guidelines on the Management of Anemia in Chronic Kidney Disease

Region	Guideline	Year of publication
US	National Kidney Foundation: DOQI Clinical Practice Guidelines for the Treatment of Anemia of Chronic Renal Failure [1]	1997
Europe	European Best Practice Guidelines [2]	1999
Canada	Canadian guidelines on anemia management [3]	1999
US	National Kidney Foundation: KDOQI Clinical Practice Guidelines for Anemia of Chronic Kidney Disease: Update 2000 [4]	2001
Europe	Revised European Best Practice Guidelines [5]	2004
Japan	Japanese guidelines on anemia management [6]	2004
Australasia	Caring for Australasians with Renal Impairment [7]	2005
UK	National Institute for Health and Clinical Excellence [8]	2006
US	KDOQI Clinical Practice Guideline and Clinical Practice Recommendations for Anemia in Chronic Kidney Disease: 2007 Update of Hemoglobin Target [9]	2007
Europe	European Best Practice Guidelines (position statement only; no new evidence review) [10]	2010
UK	National Institute for Health and Clinical Excellence (update) [11]	2011
Global	KDIGO Clinical Practice Guideline for Anemia in Chronic Kidney Disease [12]	2012

Table 8.1 Clinical Practice Guidelines on the Management of Anemia in Chronic Kidney Disease. DOQI, Disease Outcomes Quality Initiative; KDIGO, Kidney Disease: Improving Global Outcomes; KDOQI, Kidney Disease Outcomes Quality Initiative.

Key points from the KDIGO 2012 Anemia Guideline

KDIGO 2012 Anemia Guideline statement	Summary
2.1.2: For adult CKD patients with anemia not on iron or ESA therapy we suggest a trial of IV iron if (2C): • an increase in Hb concentration without starting ESA treatment is desired, and • TSAT is ≤30% and ferritin is ≤500 µg/L	Do NOT start ESA in ND CKD patients with Hb >10 g/dL
3.4.1: For CKD ND patients with Hb ≥10.0 g/dL, we suggest that ESA therapy not be initiated (2D)	
3.4.2: For CKD ND patients with Hb <10.0 g/dL, we suggest that the decision whether to initiate ESA therapy be individualized based on the rate of fall of Hb, the risk of needing a transfusion, the risks related to ESA therapy, and the presence of symptoms attributable to anemia (2C)	Start ESA if a ND CKD patient with Hb <10 g/dL is iron-replete and there is a likelihood of Hb falling below 9 g/dL

Table 8.2 Key points from the KDIGO 2012 Anemia Guideline (continues opposite).

Key points from the KDIGO 2012 Anemia Guideline (continued)

KDIGO 2012 Anemia Guideline statement	Summary
3.4.3: For CKD 5D patients, we suggest that ESA therapy be used to avoid having the Hb concentration fall below 9.0 g/dL by starting ESA therapy when the hemoglobin is between 9.0 and 10.0 g/dL (2B)	Start ESA therapy in a patient on dialysis with Hb of 9 or 10 g/dL
3.5.1: In general, we suggest that ESAs not be used to maintain Hb concentration above 11.5 g/dL (115 g/L) in adult patients with CKD (2C)	ESA should not be used to intentionally increase the Hb >13 g/dL
3.5.2: Individualization of therapy will be necessary as some patients may have improvements in quality of life at Hb concentration above 11.5 g/dL (115 g/L) and will be prepared to accept the risks (Not graded)	
3.6: In all adult patients, we recommend that ESAs not be used to intentionally increase the Hb concentration above 13 g/dL (130 g/L) (1A)	

Table 8.2 Key points from the KDIGO 2012 Anemia Guideline (continued). 5D, chronic kidney disease stage 5; CKD, chronic kidney disease; ESA, erythropoiesis-stimulating agent; Hb, hemoglobin; KDIGO, Kidney Disease: Improving Global Outcomes; ND, nondialysis; TSAT, transferrin saturation.

Key points from ERBP position statement

- Hb target should generally be 11 to 12 g/dL, not intentionally exceeding 13 g/dL
- Target Hb is only applicable to ESA therapy, not iron therapy or no treatment
- The trigger for starting ESA therapy is Hb 10 to 11 g/dL
- Doses of ESA are important; use lowest doses possible and avoid high doses of ESA
- Exercise caution using ESA therapy in patients with previous stroke or malignancy
- Consider risk : benefit of transfusions in potential transplant recipients
- Individualize therapy
- Patient's opinion should be considered

Table 8.3 Key points from ERBP position statement. ERBP, European Renal Best Practice; ESA, erythropoiesis-stimulating agent; Hb, hemoglobin. Based on data from Locatelli et al [10].

References

1 NKF-DOQI Clinical Practice Guidelines for the Treatment of Anemia of Chronic Renal Failure. National Kidney Foundation-Dialysis Outcomes Quality Initiative. *Am J Kidney Dis*. 1997;30(suppl 3):S192-S240.
2 Cameron JS. European Best Practice Guidelines for the Management of Anaemia in Patients with Chronic Renal Failure. *Nephrol Dial Transplant*. 1999;14(suppl 2):61-65.
3 Barrett BJ, Fenton SS, Ferguson B, et al. Clinical practice guidelines for the management of anemia coexistent with chronic renal failure. Canadian Society of Nephrology. *J Am Soc Nephrol*. 1999;10(suppl 13):S292-S296.
4 NKF-K/DOQI Clinical Practice Guidelines for Anemia of Chronic Kidney Disease: update 2000. *Am J Kidney Dis*. 2001;37(suppl 1):S182-S238.

5   Locatelli F, Aljama P, Bárány P, et al. Revised European best practice guidelines for the management of anaemia in patients with chronic renal failure. *Nephrol Dial Transplant.* 2004;19(suppl 2):ii1-47.

6   Gejyo F, Saito A, Akizawa T, et al. 2004 Japanese Society for Dialysis Therapy guidelines for renal anemia in chronic hemodialysis patients. *Ther Apher Dial.* 2004;8:443-459.

7   Pollock C, McMahon L. The CARI guidelines. Biochemical and haematological targets guidelines. Haemoglobin. *Nephrology (Carlton).* 2005;10(suppl 4):S108-S115.

8   National Institute for Health and Clinical Excellence. Anaemia management in people with chronic kidney disease. www.nice.org.uk/CG039. Updated March 2012. Accessed February 6, 2013.

9   National Kidney Foundation. KDOQI clinical practice guideline and clinical practice recommendations for anemia in chronic kidney disease: 2007 update of hemoglobin target. *Am J Kidney Dis.* 2007;50:471-530.

10 Locatelli F, Aljama P, Canaud B, et al. Target haemoglobin to aim for with erythropoiesis-stimulating agents: a position statement by ERBP following publication of the trial to reduce cardiovascular events with Aranesp therapy (TREAT) study. *Nephrol Dial Transplant.* 2010;25:2846-2850.

11 National Institute for Health and Clinical Excellence. Anaemia management in people with chronic kidney disease. http://guidance.nice.org.uk/CG114. Updated November 2012. Accessed February 6, 2013.

12 National Kidney Foundation. KDIGO clinical practice guideline for anemia in chronic kidney disease. *Kidney Int Suppl.* 2012;2:v-335.

Development of this book was supported by funding from Amgen

Chapter 9

What is the future of renal anemia management?

As detailed in chapters 5, 6, and 7, the mainstay of anemia management includes ESA therapy, iron management, and blood transfusions [1]. ESA therapy has evolved from a recombinant protein to a hyperglycosylated molecule, to a pegylated protein, to an erythropoietin-mimetic peptide. However, all of these developments have in common the fact that the molecule binds to the erythropoietin receptor and induces a common intracellular signaling cascade, which ultimately leads to the enhanced survival and proliferation of primitive erythroid cells.

Several newer strategies are under development, and the reader is directed to a recent comprehensive review [2]. Two novel strategies, HIF stabilization and hepcidin modulation, are worthy of mention, particularly as both are in clinical trials and could therefore potentially become licensed therapeutic agents within the next few years.

Hypoxia-inducible factor stabilizers

HIF is the major transcription factor for the erythropoietin gene (see Figure 2.2). It is broken down by a prolyl hydroxylase enzyme, and orally active inhibitors of this enzyme have now been synthesized. Inhibition of prolyl hydroxylase stabilizes the HIF molecule (similar to what happens physiologically at high altitude), and HIF is then able to bind to the hypoxia-responsive element of the erythropoietin gene to upregulate erythropoietin synthesis. Thus, instead of patients requiring to have injections of recombinant erythropoietin or one of its analogs, patients

I. C. Macdougall, *Pocket Reference to Renal Anemia*,
DOI: 10.1007/978-1-907673-48-1_9, © Springer Healthcare 2013

are stimulated to produce their own erythropoietin. This mechanism is effective even in end-stage renal disease [3] and, even more remarkably, in anephric individuals in whom the erythropoietin is believed to be synthesized in the liver [3].

A number of candidate HIF stabilizer molecules are in Phase I, II, and III clinical trials, and these agents may potentially be administered once-daily or three times a week. The main advantage of this strategy, if successful, would be the ability to use orally active agents to enhance erythropoietin activity, as all currently available ESAs are injectable therapies. One potential limitation of this strategy is that there are many other genes (well over 100) that are hypoxia-sensitive, and may also be upregulated by stabilization of HIF. Other genes that potentially could be upregulated include those involved in angiogenesis, gluconeogenesis, and connective tissue synthesis. Liver toxicity was also a problem with the first-generation molecule (FG-2216) [4], but the newer molecules would appear to be less hepatotoxic.

Hepcidin modulation

As discussed earlier, hepcidin is critically involved in iron regulation in the body. It controls how much dietary iron is absorbed from the gut, and also how much iron is released from the reticuloendothelial system where it is normally stored (see Figure 2.5). In conditions of active inflammation, hepcidin synthesis is increased (largely through stimulation by IL-6) [5], and this will cause trapping of iron in the cells of the reticuloendothelial system. This, in turn, will exacerbate anemia by restricting iron availability to the bone marrow.

Inhibiting hepcidin activity, therefore, is a potential novel approach to treating anemia in inflammatory conditions such as CKD. This has been put to the test in a mouse model of inflammation, using a monoclonal antibody against hepcidin [6]. Although, as a proof of concept, this strategy was effective in this animal model, this is potentially a cumbersome and costly means of treating anemia. Many other strategies are currently being explored, being broadly divided into those that antagonize hepcidin or its action, and those that inhibit hepcidin synthesis [7]. Whether any such agents would be effective on their own, or as an adjunct to erythropoietin stimulation, is unclear at the present time. It would seem likely that the requirements for supplemental iron would be less with hepcidin antagonism, as absorption of dietary iron would be increased.

Other strategies

Other strategies such as GATA-2 inhibition [8] and erythropoietin gene therapy [9] are also being explored. Inhibition of GATA-2 acts in a similar way to HIF stabilization, as GATA-2 is inhibitory to erythropoietin gene transcription. Thus, antagonizing this transcription factor produces upregulation of the erythropoietin gene.

The first of the erythropoietin gene therapies is currently in Phase II clinical trials [10]. This strategy involves a microdermal biopsy of the skin, harvesting the skin cells, and then transfecting them with the erythropoietin gene. The cells are then implanted back into the forearm of the patient, allowing ongoing synthesis of endogenous erythropoietin. Several patients have now been maintained for more than 1 year using this strategy.

References

1   National Kidney Foundation. KDIGO clinical practice guideline for anemia in chronic kidney disease. *Kidney Int Suppl*. 2012;2:v-335.
2   Macdougall IC. New anemia therapies: translating novel strategies from bench to bedside. *Am J Kidney Dis*. 2012;59:444-451.
3   Bernhardt WM, Wiesener MS, Scigalla P, et al. Inhibition of prolyl hydroxylases increases erythropoietin production in ESRD. *J Am Soc Nephrol*. 2010;21:2151-2156.
4   Astellas Pharma Inc. Adverse event of FG-2216 for the treatment of anemia. Media Release May 07, 2007. http://www.astellas.com/en/corporate/news/pdf/070507_eg.pdf. Accessed February 6, 2013.
5   Nemeth E, Rivera S, Gabayan V, et al. IL-6 mediates hypoferremia of inflammation by inducing the synthesis of the iron regulatory hormone hepcidin. *J Clin Invest*. 2004;113:1271-1276.
6   Sasu BJ, Cooke KS, Arvedson TL, et al. Antihepcidin antibody treatment modulates iron metabolism and is effective in a mouse model of inflammation-induced anemia. *Blood*. 2010;115:3616-3624.
7   Sun CC, Vaja V, Babitt JL, Lin HY. Targeting the hepcidin-ferroportin axis to develop new treatment strategies for anemia of chronic disease and anemia of inflammation. *Am J Hematol*. 2012;87:392-400.
8   Imagawa S, Yamamoto M, Miura Y. Negative regulation of the erythropoietin gene expression by the GATA transcription factors. *Blood*. 1997;89:1430-1439.

9 Brill-Almon E, Stern B, Afik D, et al. Ex vivo transduction of human dermal tissue structures for autologous implantation production and delivery of therapeutic proteins. *Mol Ther.* 2005;12:274-282.

10 Epodure therapy of anemia in end stage renal disease on dialysis with Epodure skin implant. Clinical Trials website. clinicaltrials.gov/ct2/show/NCT01555515?term=EPODURE&rank=2. Accessed February 6, 2013.

Development of this book was supported by funding from Amgen

Chapter 10

Conclusions

Anemia management in CKD has seen many changes over the last few decades. Prior to 1990, the mainstay of treatment was blood transfusions and/or iron supplementation. The introduction of ESA therapy in 1990 led to a dramatic reduction in the use of RBC transfusions, while iron supplementation was instituted more widely in order to maximize the response to ESAs (as well as to keep the doses and costs as low as possible). The results from the TREAT study have strongly influenced the latest thoughts regarding anemia management, and although ESA therapy is still of critical importance in this condition, a more conservative strategy has since been recommended. The logical stepwise approach to renal anemia management remains as: (i) exclusion of any other contributory cause of anemia; (ii) iron management; (iii) ESA therapy; and (iv) blood transfusions. Finally, other strategies for treating anemia in CKD are currently being researched, including hepcidin modulation strategies and HIF stabilization by prolyl hydroxylase inhibitors. It is too early to say what role these new scientific developments will have in the management of CKD anemia, but they are certainly of academic interest and worthy of further investigation.

I. C. Macdougall, *Pocket Reference to Renal Anemia*,
DOI: 10.1007/978-1-907673-48-1_10, © Springer Healthcare 2013

Dos and don'ts in renal anemia management

Do

- Do use IV iron first when possible, especially if ferritin is <100 µg/L
- Do start ESA therapy when Hb levels are 9–10 g/dL rather than 10–11 g/dL
- Do aim for a target of Hb of 10–12 g/dL
- Do consider risk–benefit ratio in patients with CKD with previous stroke or cancer

Don't

- Do *not* escalate ESA dose in patients responding poorly to treatment
- Do *not* administer IV iron to patients with active infection

Learning points

Learning point 1
Renal anemia usually occurs when the GFR falls below 30 mL/min, although mild degrees of anemia may be present with a GFR of up to 60 mL/min [1].

Learning point 2
Diabetics appear to develop inappropriately low levels of erythropoietin at a higher GFR cut-off compared to nondiabetics. Thus it is not uncommon for diabetic subjects to develop renal anemia when their GFR falls below 45 mL/min [2].

Learning point 3
In healthy individuals, the bone marrow manufactures approximately 120 million new RBCs every minute.

Learning point 4
CKD patients in stages 1, 2, and early stage 3 who are found to be anemic, require stringent investigations for other causes of anemia, as renal anemia alone is much less likely [1].

Learning point 5
"Pure" renal anemia is usually normochromic and normocytic, and either a low or high MCV, or low MCH or MCHC strongly suggest other contributory causes.

Learning point 6
A low MCV commonly occurs in patients receiving sirolimus therapy [3].

Learning point 7
A low MCV coupled with a low MCH or MCHC indicates either iron deficiency or a hemoglobinopathy.

Learning point 8
A rapid change in MCV and/or RBC volume distribution width strongly suggest that the patient has had a recent RBC transfusion.

Learning point 9
A reticulocyte count of $<10 \times 10^9$/L suggests severe bone marrow failure, possibly due to antibody-mediated pure red cell aplasia or another hematological condition [4].

Learning point 10
Reticulocyte counts of $>100 \times 10^9$/L suggest an active bone marrow, but enhanced RBC loss, due to either hemolysis or bleeding.

Learning point 11
A very low serum ferritin level (eg, <20 µg/L), conclusively proves a diagnosis of absolute iron deficiency, as there is no other cause for such a low level.

Learning point 12
Serum iron on its own is unhelpful as an indicator of iron deficiency, but its relationship to the total iron-binding capacity, expressed as a percentage (transferrin saturation) may be useful.

Learning point 13
IV iron should not be given to patients with acute bacterial infection.

Learning point 14
The trigger hemoglobin concentration for initiating ESA therapy should be somewhere around 9 or 10 g/dL, with the aim of preventing patients' hemogolobin levels from falling below 9 g/dL [5].

Learning point 15
The target hemoglobin concentration for patients receiving ESA therapy should be individualized, but should be somewhere around 10–12 g/dL [6].

Learning point 16
In patients showing a suboptimal response to ESA therapy, the reticulocyte count may provide helpful information. If low, then erythropoiesis is probably suppressed or deficient, whereas a high reticulocyte count might suggest bleeding or hemolysis.

Learning point 17
In the absence of acute bleeding, there is little indication to transfuse a patient with hemoglobil levels above 7 or 8 g/dL unless a surgical procedure is planned in which significant blood loss might be expected [5].

References

1 Astor BC, Muntner P, Levin A, et al. Association of kidney function with anemia: the Third National Health and Nutrition Examination Survey (1988–1994). *Arch Intern Med*. 2002;162:1401-1408.
2 Thomas MC, MacIsaac RJ, Tsalamandris C, Power D, Jerums G. Unrecognized anemia in patients with diabetes: a cross-sectional survey. *Diabetes Care*. 2003;26:1164-1169.

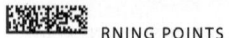 RNING POINTS

3   Thaunat O, Beaumont C, Chatenoud L, et al. Anemia after late introduction of sirolimus may correlate with biochemical evidence of a chronic inflammatory state. *Transplantation*. 2005;80:1212-1219.

4   Pollock C, Johnson DW, Hörl WH, et al. Pure red cell aplasia induced by erythropoiesis-stimulating agents. *Clin J Am Soc Nephrol*. 2008;3:193-199.

5   National Kidney Foundation. KDIGO clinical practice guideline for anemia in chronic kidney disease. *Kidney Int Suppl*. 2012;2:v-335.

6   National Institute for Health and Clinical Excellence. Anaemia management in people with chronic kidney disease. http://guidance.nice.org.uk/CG114. Updated November 2012. Accessed February 6, 2013.

Development of this book was supported by funding from Amgen